Vagus Nerve Healing

Improve Your Immune System, Overcome Brain Fog, Inflammations, and Digestive Disorders with Self Help Exercises for Vagus Nerve Stimulation. Help for Anxiety and Depression.

Dr. Louise Lily Wain

All effort has been executed to present accurate, up to date, and reliable, complete information. No warranties of any kind are declared or implied.

Readers acknowledge that the author is not engaging in the rendering of legal, financial, medical or professional advice.

The content within this book has been derived from various sources.

Please consult a licensed professional before attempting any techniques outlined in this book.

By reading this document, the reader agrees that under no circumstances is the author responsible for any losses, direct or indirect, which are incurred as a result of the use of the information contained within this document, including, but not limited to, — errors, omissions, or inaccuracies.

Table of Contents

Chapter 12: The Vagus Nerve and Other Common Conditions 180

Conclusion 187
List of Books written by Dr. Louise Lily Wain 189

Introduction

Congratulations on purchasing *Vagus Nerve Healing,* and thank you for doing so.

Most people know that the brain is the ultimate regulator of the body—but they do not usually know why.

Each and every person has a pair of nerves in their bodies that go from the brainstem all the way down throughout most of the abdomen, all the way through to the digestive tract.

This particular set of cranial nerves is the longest of the body, and it reaches out to every major organ that you have.

It controls and influences your ability to speak.

It influences whether or not you will respond to danger with panic or anger.

It determines how you will act around other people.

It can influence your heart rate.

It can make you want to sleep. It can even make you faint in certain situations.

It can paralyze the stomach, or it can ease inflammation.

It can regulate appetite while also encouraging feelings of happiness.

This one nerve acts as a sort of ultimate regulator of the body, allowing for all sorts of different functions to occur, and many times, people completely neglect to realize that it is there.

This nerve is your vagus nerve—the vagabond nerve that is able to travel throughout all of your body and regulate it all in many ways.

This nerve acts as a sort of direct channel of communication between your important visceral organs and the brain so it can all be regulated quickly and efficiently.

By cutting out the middle-man of the spine, which normally acts as that sort of translator for the body to the brain, signals can be sent quicker, easier, and more efficiently than ever.

This very same nerve is also capable of great things.

Thanks to how big it is and the areas that it travels throughout the body, it is able to regulate just about anything.

It can be directly stimulated to allow for the activation of this nerve, through touch, sound, and even indirectly.

There are many ways that you can make use of this yourself.

However, sometimes, such an important nerve can malfunction, so to speak.

It can stop working as efficiently as it should be, and when that happens, you run into a very simple problem—your body is not going to work the way that it should be.

People can find that they are more anxious than necessary—and it could be a problem with the vagus nerve.

Depression could be linked to it, as well.

Many inflammation-related disorders have also been treated through the use of stimulation of the vagus nerve, and because of that, it is very quickly gaining attention from all over the world.

When you make use of stimulating your vagus nerve yourself, you can help your body regulate itself out.

You can help the body become healthier than ever—you can ensure that, at the end of the day, your body will be more capable of regulating itself out.

You can almost guarantee that your body is going to be able to work more efficiently because you are toning up your vagus nerve, which will allow it to better regulate your body.

This book is here to teach you to do precisely that—in reading this book, you are going to learn all about how you can make better use of your vagus nerve.

You are going to learn about what it is and how it works.

You are going to be introduced to how you can check on whether or not your own vagus nerve is toned and able to regulate your body, or if it is likely to be causing problems for you.

You will learn how you can then work to stimulate and tone your own vagus nerve.

This does not have to be invasive or require surgery—there are some devices that your doctor may eventually recommend for you to use, but for the most part, you can stimulate your vagus nerve at home with ease.

All that you have to do is know where in the body it is so you can then make good use of several activities and techniques that will stimulate it.

These activities will be given to you in the last half of the book.

As we address common problems that the vagus nerve can cause, we will also look at two ways that you can stimulate or tone your vagus nerve at home so you can help mitigate the problem to the best of your ability.

When you can do this, you know that you are able to better cope with just about any problems that your vagus nerve may throw your way.

You will be able to help yourself get out of that panic attack with these methods or to help alleviate some of your own inflammation that you are feeling.

Ultimately, with the use of these particular methods that you will be introduced to, you should be able to bring yourself to feel better.

You will feel happier, healthier, and more in control of your body, and because you are giving yourself back the control that you may feel like you have lost, you may find that you will feel deeply satisfied in the process of doing so.

And with that said, let's take a look at how to begin understanding and working with your vagus nerve.

As you read, you will be surprised to see just how involved this one set of nerves is throughout your entire body.

Chapter 1: What Is the Vagus Nerve?

Before it is time to delve into looking at common problems with the vagus nerve, it is first imperative that you understand what the nerve is in the first place.

In this chapter, we are going to take some time to do just that.

Ultimately, your entire body is filled with nerve bundles—they can be found just about anywhere in the body, and for good reason.

Your nerves, made up of neurons that are throughout your entire body, are there to allow your brain to control it.

They are like wires on a network that will bring signals everywhere—they are mapped together to allow the entire system to work together.

They allow messages to go from your brain to the tip of your toes and back again nearly instantaneously and without effort on your part.

Within this chapter, we are going to take some time to understand the nerves themselves.

We are going to look at the nerves and how they work.

Then, we are going to take a look at the nervous system and how it can be used to function accordingly.

Then, we will take a look at the cranial nerves throughout the system and see what jobs they hold.

Finally, we will get to the vagus nerve—a very important nerve that is responsible for the regulation of most of your organs.

In understanding this background information, you will be able to better appreciate and understand the rest of this book and how all of these parts can sort of intermingling, connecting and interacting with each other, even if the parts may seem unrelated at first.

Understanding Nerves

Nerves are the fundamental building block of the nervous system.

These are bundles of neurons—the individual nerve cells—that come together to allow for messages to be sent from place to place.

Think, for a moment, about how children play a game of telephone.

The message goes from one child to the next, and from that child to the next one, so on until it reaches the proper ending point.

The children are acting as a sort of network with several points when they do this—they are passing a message from place to place to place, repeating the message to the next person in the chain.

This is the same concept that gets used by your nerves.

However, nerves do this on a much larger scale.

The nerves will pass a message from neuron to neuron, from one part of the body until they reach the ending point elsewhere.

This is important—it is how the body communicates with the brain as well as how the brain is able to communicate with the body.

Each nerve has two ends—it has the receiving end and the sending end.

These ends come together, nestled into each other.

It is where they connect to each other that they are able to pass their messages along from one spot to the next.

This is done in two ways—electrically and chemically.

Nerves communicate through what is known as an electrochemical system.

Let's say that you poke your finger on something sharp.

When that happens, the local nerves in the area receive the message.

They send "SHARP!" down their axons—the long, skinny portion of the cell.

This is done through an electrical impulse.

The electrical impulse is sent all the way down the axon to the end of the neuron, where it is connected to many more neurons at that point.

The message is then translated from "SHARP" in electrical impulses to a chemical one.

The neuron then sends that chemical message across to the next neuron, which reads the message and then sends another electrical impulse of "SHARP!"

This will happen repeatedly, mapping across neurons, and each one can connect to upwards of a thousand more.

The message then gets shot through your body—in some areas, roughly at 120 miles per second in speed to get to the brain.

The fastest nerve of all—the alpha motor neuron in the spinal cord, is able to transmit messages at speeds of over 260 mph to your brain.

When you consider just how small the body is, as well as the scale of how small these neurons would be, this is nearly instantaneous—this is why you feel something just about immediately upon it happening.

Your nerves serve one of two purposes—they will either send signals back to the brain that was received through a sense— they are afferent nerves.

Other nerves will send signals from the brain to the body—these are efferent nerves.

Some nerves, such as the vagus nerve, can do a bit of both process, making them capable of much more than the average nerve that they are going to have access to.

The Nervous System

All of those nerves that you have in your body are all able to come together into what is known as the nervous system.

Your nervous system is the system of neurons within your body, and it is commonly thought of in terms of hierarchies to allow it to be understood by purpose.

Each nervous system that we are going over will serve a slightly different purpose.

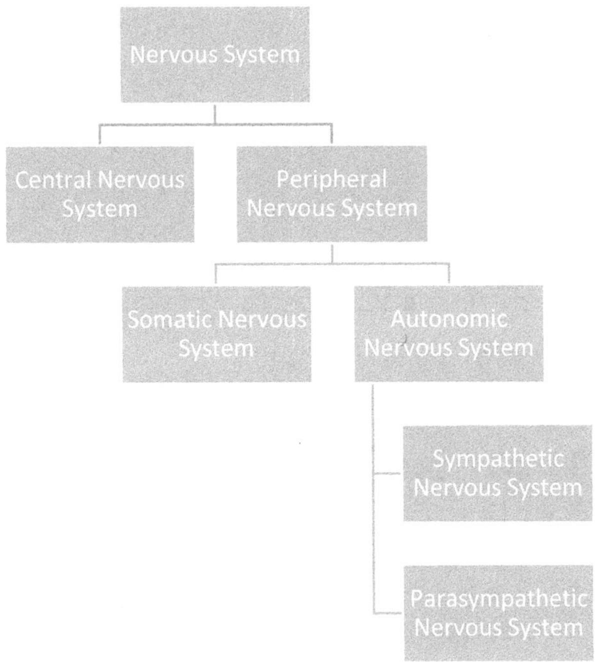

Central and peripheral nervous systems

The first divide to understand is the central and peripheral nervous system.

The central nervous system is the primary processing power of your body.

This is your brain and the spinal cord connected to it.

This part of your nervous system does all of the processing to allow your body to function at the end of the day.

Your brain is responsible for the vast majority of the processing, but the spinal cord is capable of some degree of processing as well—particularly when it comes to reflexes.

Your spinal cord I sable to handle these reflexes, which is why they happen nearly instantaneously and involuntarily—they happen on their own due to the spine.

Everything that is not your spine or your brain is your central nervous system.

This means that any nerves anywhere else in your body will be considered peripheral.

This includes your vagus nerve—as a cranial nerve, these nerves travel from the brain elsewhere into the body, but they are not a part of the spine or the brain, making them technically a peripheral part of the system.

The peripheral nervous system is how your body is able to interact with the world around it. It will include several different parts to it as well.

Autonomic vs. somatic nervous system

The peripheral nervous system is commonly divided further—it gets divided into the autonomic and the somatic nervous systems.

Your somatic nervous system is a bit simpler, so we will consider this one first.

This is the part of the nervous system that is responsible for carrying sensory information.

It collects all of that sensory data and ensures that it gets to where it needs to be, to be understood by other parts of the body as well.

This is a very important job—without it, your body would not be able to react and respond to the rest of the world.

It also includes motor commands to the muscles that you have.

This is your set of voluntary controls over your body.

Anything that you do that is voluntary will be a part of your peripheral nervous system.

Your autonomic nervous system, however, is the involuntary part of your body's regulation.

This is responsible for controlling all of those involuntary processes that will keep you alive.

You cannot, for example, will your heart to stop.

While you could control how much you are breathing when conscious, your body will blackout before it is able to truly be deprived of oxygen—at which point it will be right back to be able to be controlled by the autonomic system.

This part of the nervous system happens on its own without any need for intervention.

This is, to some degree, to allow for instantaneous functionality without having to be consciously aware of it at all times.

Your autonomic nervous system gets divided even further.

Sympathetic and parasympathetic nervous systems

The autonomic nervous system is then broken down further into the sympathetic and parasympathetic nervous systems.

These allow for your body to regulate itself out in different ways.

Generally speaking, your parasympathetic nervous system is going to be responsible for calming you down—it will encourage your body to rest and digest.

It wants your body to conserve energy for future use when it activates.

This is important—you cannot digest food properly if you are stuck without this particular nervous system capable of engaging.

Your body needs this to cope with stress, should stress occur at any point in time.

The sympathetic nervous system is the opposite—it encourages arousal and alertness in the body.

Usually, this is attributed to fear—it encourages the body to pay closer attention than ever to the surroundings.

When you are in a state of sympathetic activation, your body is not going to respond well to the world around it. It is going to be focusing on staying alive, typically in response to some sort of stress.

You will see high levels of agitation or nervousness during this activation, and that can be a huge problem for you.

Your body ultimately is designed to spend most of its time in a parasympathetic state—with this state; you are calm and relaxed.

While the sympathetic reaction has a very important job, it is also not very healthy to be kept in for an extended period of time.

When you worry about that, you then see that the individual is likely to struggle with stress and anxiety.

They may be agitated and angry.

They may find that they do not want to get along with other people.

Cranial Nerves

Before we get to the vagus nerve and where it sits within the nervous system, however, let's stop and consider what cranial nerves are for a moment—these nerves are very special within the body—there are only twelve pairs within the body.

However, they all serve very important purposes within the body.

These are nerves that are able to bypass the spinal cord.

The vast majority of nerves throughout the body go straight through the spinal cord.

However, the cranial nerves are exceptions to this rule.

They are directly connected to the brain—they all connect right around the brainstem and go straight down into the body.

Most of these are paired up around the face—they are responsible for controlling the special senses in the sensory organs in the face.

These are responsible for actions such as being able to sense smell or taste.

The vagus nerve is a bit of an exception to this—while it does provide a small degree of sensory input for the sensory organs, it is primarily concentrated in the visceral organs, as we will be addressing shortly.

The Vagus Nerve

The vagus nerve is a very special nerve. It is the longest of the cranial nerves—it goes from the brainstem all the way down throughout the digestive system.

It has several very specific functions as well that are quite unique to it alone.

In particular, it is responsible for general somatic sensory abilities—this is its ability to return information to the brain about the senses that it is able to receive from the ear, from the larynx, and from the pharynx.

It is involved in your ability to speak and your sense of balance.

It is also responsible for general visceral sensory information—it connects to several of the organs within your chest and abdomen.

In particular, it connects to the lungs, the heart, and just about all of the digestive tracts.

This nerve is both efferent and afferent—it is able to not only provide sensory input for the brain to process and use, but it is also able to provide some degree of movement as well.

In particular, the vagus nerve controls some of the movements of the vocal cords as well as the digestive system.

It also is responsible for allowing for a sense of taste—specifically from the back of the tongue.

This makes it incredibly versatile.

After all, most people would not say that the intestines, the heart, the lungs, and the tongue all should involve the same wiring—but to some degree, they do!

This is precisely why the vagus nerve is so unique, to begin with—it involves several different areas of the body and is in

control of many of the ones that will keep people alive at the end
of the day.

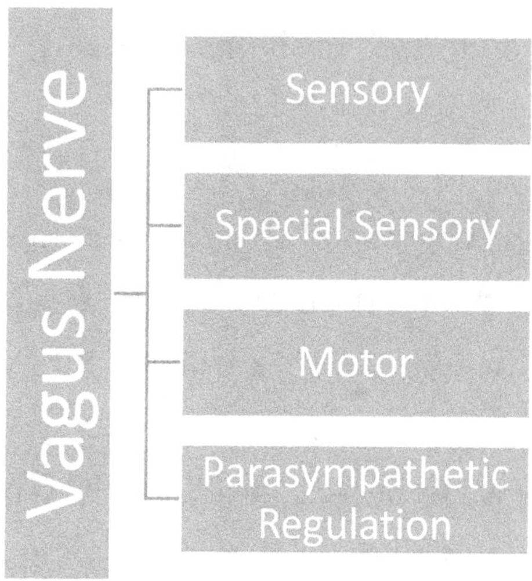

Generally speaking, the vagus nerve has four key functions that
must occur in order to allow it to work properly. These are:

- **Sensory functions:** The vagus nerve is responsible for
  providing sensory data throughout the body.

  It gathers up most of the important data from the throat,
  heart, lungs, and vital organs to send up to the brain for
  future processing.

It does this entirely unconsciously, but it is what allows your brain to determine all sorts of information about the status of your organs at any given point in time.

It will allow, for example, your brain to tell your stomach that it needs to feel hungry now.

It does this so you are able to regulate out blood sugar and how much food your system can process at any point in time.

You may not feel that sensation of food in your gut or how it feels for it to travel throughout the digestive system, but the vagus nerve is paying attention to it and ensuring that it all gets passed through accordingly.

- **Special sensory functions:** This is the use of any of the senses that you have.

  In special senses, you are able to relate to what you are doing at any point in time.

  This will allow you to sense the world around you.

  The vagus nerve, in particular, is in control of the sense of taste at the base of your tongue.

- **Motor functions:** This is the ability to move and control your body.

  The vagus nerve controls the muscles inside of your neck that are commonly used in speaking and swallowing.

- **Parasympathetic regulation:** This is the ability to control the parasympathetic nervous system.

  The vagus nerve, in particular, is in complete control of this system.

  It can make the strength of your parasympathetic system weaker or stronger, and by default in doing so, it is able to help regulate out the sympathetic nervous system as well, giving it that position as a sort of autonomic regulator in general.

Chapter 2: The Vagus Nerve, the Autonomic Nervous System, and Regulation

The vagus nerve, with all of the reach, that it has throughout the body is capable of making you feel some pretty strong feelings at any point in time.

This makes sense if you think about it—if it can control so many areas in your body, from your pulse to your blood pressure to the way that your stomach is feeling, it should be capable of making your body feel a certain way as well.

You will, in particular, be able to have very visceral responses to your vagus nerve just due to the fact that it does have so much control over your body.

Think about it for a moment—when you are angry and trying not to lose your cool, what do you do?

You probably take a big, deep breath, right?

The reason you do this is that your body is able to activate the vagus nerve in response.

You take in a breath that involves the pressure within your chest changing—you drop the pressure in your chest to allow for the air to be sucked inward.

The vagus nerve responds to that change in pressure by changing the blood pressure rate and the pulse rate—those get knocked down to accommodate accordingly to allow for the body to then regulate itself out.

When you exhale, you raise the pressure in your chest to allow for the air to be squeezed out, and in response, your body will then trigger the vagus nerve.

The vagus nerve activates when you exhale by lowering your pulse to drop blood pressure to regulate out with the pressure that is felt in your chest.

Essentially, the body regulates itself out at all times to try to keep itself as close to homeostasis as possible, and it does this in the ways that it is able to interact with the body.

This means that if you can interfere with other parts of your body, you can also encourage other parts of your body to then activate the vagus nerve indirectly.

This is great—it is what allows your body to really function the way that it does.

Because it is a big balancing act to regulate it all out, your body has its own built-in control system if you know how to alter certain readings within it.

Within this chapter, we are going to address the ways in which your vagus nerve activates in your body.

We are taking a look in particular at how the vagus nerve acts as a sort of regulator.

It regulates your responses in many different ways—it controls your reaction to stress.

It activates either your sympathetic or parasympathetic responses.

It allows you to regulate most of the functions of your body.

We are going to take a look at the vagus nerve in these contexts to allow for a better understanding of what it does and how it works.

If you can get that understanding down, you will then be able to begin making use of controlling your own vagus nerve in many different situations.

The Vagus Nerve and Stress

The vagus nerve primarily responds to stress within the body.

It is constantly watching what is going on in your body—it is paying attention to your heart rate and lung capacity.

It is paying attention to how full your stomach is and what your blood sugar is at.

It is able to regulate all of this and more thanks to how far it reaches out.

However, what its primary job actually is, is the ability to regulate the stress response.

In particular, you will find that your vagus nerve is particularly responsive to stress.

Have you ever fainted when something scared you?

Perhaps you saw blood, and suddenly, you were waking up on the ground.

Maybe you know someone who has been there before.

If that sounds familiar to you, you are thinking of someone, or yourself, having a *vasovagal* response.

Look at that root word there—vagal.

This is because the vagus nerve is involved.

Fainting, most of the time is caused by your body's overreaction in the face of stress.

Your vagus nerve is supposed to sort of regulate whether you should keep calm or blow up on other people.

It takes a look at how the body is going to respond in the face of stress.

It will most of the time act to regulate the system—it will try to keep you calm.

It does this by activating to send out parasympathetic signals.

This tells your body to calm down when it senses that you are getting stressed out.

However, sometimes, it *over*reacts, and it causes your blood pressure to suddenly plummet.

Without enough blood pressure to get blood up to your brain, you suddenly lose consciousness—you faint.

This happened because your body overreacted to the stress of whatever it was that you had seen.

The vagus nerve acts as a sort of regulator of whether or not you are going to be stressed out by something.

If it sees the problem as something worthy of the stress response in the first place, it will respond by releasing the parasympathetic response—it will sort of mute that response that normally keeps the sympathetic nervous system under control and it will let the sympathetic nervous system activate, leading to your stress response.

The Vagus Nerve and Sympathetic Activation

Sympathetic activation is a state in which your body has allowed the sympathetic response to rule.

This happens when the vagus nerve mutes the parasympathetic response that will normally be controlled by the vagus nerve.

When the parasympathetic response gets turned off, your body is going to immediately go into a sympathetic response by default.

When this happens, your body will face a stress response.

This will prep your body for one of two responses—you can fight, or you can flee.

Your body is trying to figure out how it is that you can escape and solve the stress as quickly as possible when this happens.

When your body is under a sympathetic activation, it will unconsciously trigger all sorts of changes to the body.

Your heart rate goes up so your body can pump more oxygen throughout your system.

Your pupils dilate, and you become a bit more responsive to the world around you.

Your temperature changes and your body shifts from being able to respond in a resting state to be focused on how to escape from whatever has stressed it out.

Usually, the digestive system turns off—it stops focusing on trying to digest food because there are more important areas that energy could go.

The body floods hormones throughout itself to allow for this extended response, encouraging the reaction even further.

As this happens, you begin to breathe rapidly to get more oxygen for your brain.

The blood gets extra glucose pumped throughout it.

Oftentimes, this happens without you realizing it—the body is incredibly skilled at honing these responses.

Think about it this way—when you are walking across the street and suddenly see a car driving right for you, you do not stop to ponder what to do next.

Your body simply makes you move.

Your fight or flight response kicks in, and you react as quickly as you can.

This then allows you to have that response time and reflex to jump out of the way before you even realize that it is happening. After the stressor is gone, however, this activation does not suddenly pass on its own.

Your body cannot get itself out of this sort of fight or flight response—it needs help to do so.

It will continue to exist in this state of increased awareness and alertness for an extended period of time if your body does not regulate itself out.

The Vagus Nerve and Parasympathetic Activation

The parasympathetic nervous system is precisely the part that will regulate that sympathetic activation.

When your body senses that the stressor is no longer an important aspect of what is happening, it will turn on and lead to the vagus nerve slowing down the body.

Instead of panicking, you will find that the vagus nerve will slow down the body and allow it to return back to that homeostasis state in which it can complete the digestive cycle without strain.

When the parasympathetic response kicks in again, it will tell the body to rest—it will slow down blood pressure and breathing rates to allow the body to adjust back to pre-stressor levels.

It will do this along with regulating out the hormone levels to allow the body to return back to that state of homeostasis.

Your body will allow itself to continue digesting food without worry.

You will feel calmer.

You will feel like you are able to relax and go to sleep if you choose to do so.

This particular state is your default state.

Without this state, you will find that you are stuck in that constant state of agitation and alertness that will prevent you from getting any real, meaningful rest.

You need your body to return to this state in order for normal functioning.

However, sometimes, the vagus nerve is not able to activate entirely when it should.

During that period of stress, sometimes, the vagus nerve never steps in to intervene.

When this happens, you run into a new problem altogether—the body does not calm down.

It continues to be inundated by the stress of the sympathetic response, which is generally quite rough on the body.

It can cause inflammation issues, anxiety, and more just due to the lack of regulation.

The Vagus Nerve and Regulation of the Body

As the sort of keeper overall homeostasis and homeostatic functions, you would imagine that the vagus nerve gets to regulate most of the body—and it does.

It can regulate several very important functions of the body.

As a ruler of the parasympathetic nervous system, the vagus nerve is responsible for:

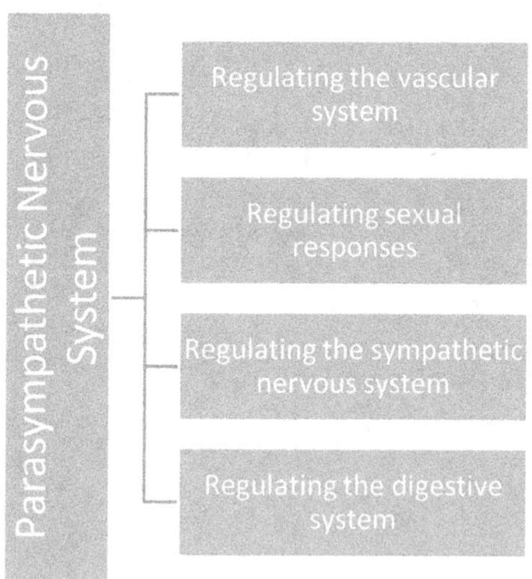

- **The vascular system:** The vagus nerve is able to regulate how quickly the heartbeats as well as the blood pressure within the body.

  It can slow it down by activating and releasing acetylcholine, or it can produce less of active response and allow the heart to beat quicker.

  Without the vagus nerve, the heart rate would be far quicker than it normally is when at rest.

- **Sexual responses:** The vagus nerve, as a regulator of the parasympathetic nervous system, gets to determine when the body is ready to reproduce.

  In fact, while the parasympathetic nervous system is associated with the "fight or flight" response, the parasympathetic response is regularly referred to as the "feed and breed" response.

- **Regulating the sympathetic nervous system:** The vagus nerve and the parasympathetic response tends to act as a sort of inhibitors over the fight or flight response of the sympathetic nervous system.

  It works sort of like the reins on a horse—when the vagus nerve is controlling the system, it is like holding the reins on the body.

However, when the vagus nerve stops, no longer activating the parasympathetic nervous system to regulate out the sympathetic one, the sympathetic response is free to run rampant—and it does.

Without the parasympathetic regulation, the body will naturally fall into this sort of stressful activation.

- **Digestion:** The vagus nerve controls much of digestion and the production of glycogen—the molecule that is used to store glucose.

  Without this, the body would not properly digest the food that needs to be taken in.

  This is directly related to the digestion control that the vagus nerve has in the first place.

Chapter 3: The Healing Power of the Vagus Nerve

Because the vagus nerve is responsible for returning the body to homeostasis, it has some degree of control over how you heal.

It can commonly be used to regulate all sorts of activations within the body—you can use your vagus nerve, for example, to aid in the regulation of the immune system and inflammation.

It pays a part in general healing by the use of stimulating it.

It is even being investigated as a genuine way to treat many different problems that people commonly suffer from, ranging from epilepsy to depression.

Within this chapter, we are going to consider precisely how the vagus nerve is able to heal so quickly and easily without much effort from other parts of the body.

We are going to be discussing how people commonly turn to the vagus nerve already to aid in their own healing, which will then allow them to better self-regulate.

Thankfully, as we will be exploring shortly, the vagus nerve does not have to be stimulated with medication or with the use of a device—you can stimulate it yourself with ease if you know what you are doing and we will be discussing precisely how to do that as you continue to read throughout this book.

Treatment does not have to be difficult—you can even just make general life changes to your current living situation, and you may be shocked to find that you can actually see some pretty significant changes to the way that you are feeling.

Keep in mind, however, that when you do want to make use of the healing power of the vagus nerve, you should never stop any sort of medically prescribed regimen.

While this can be great to help you and it can absolutely aid in many common problems that people have, ranging from their anxiety and depression all the way to their epilepsy, if you do have medication for any of the ailments that will be discussed within this book, you must remember to talk to your doctor before making a change.

Remember that the human body is complex—if you are already taking medication, you should continue to do so unless your doctor agrees that you should stop taking it.

Within this chapter, we are going to take a look at the role of the vagus nerve in the immune system, discovering what it does in terms of inflammation and the role that it plays when your body does trigger an immune response.

This can help shed some light on how this particular treatment has been being used for people that are currently suffering from autoimmune disorders.

We will take a look at how you can heal yourself, mind, and body, with the use of many of these methods.

We will look at the vagus nerve and how it is currently being used to treat both epilepsy and depression.

The Vagus Nerve and the Immune System

Despite the fact that the vagus nerve itself has nothing to do with properly patching up an injury, it does play a major role in regulating the response.

Remember, the vagus nerve is very inhibitory—it prevents things from happening.

It slows the heart.

It encourages relaxation.

It stops the sympathetic response.

It also stops inflammation.

Inflammation is a major part of the immune system—it is a part of the normal immune response and must be treated as such to allow for a proper understanding of the role that the vagus nerve will play in this all.

Inflammation is the first response to any sort of injury or any sort of illness that the body contracts.

When you get injured, your body immediately responds to it by sending out inflammation to sort of protecting the area.

This will create an area of the body that appears read and warm to the touch, and it will probably also be somewhat stiff and painful, especially if on a joint.

When your body triggers inflammation, you are going to go through six steps:

- Inflammation
- Macrophage deployment
- Blood vessels dilating
- Dendritic cells arriving
- Immune system's response with antibodies
- Recovery

The inflammation that occurs happens because the body sends extra blood to the area—it wants the area to be protected from any sort of illness, so it sends extra blood to bring with it extra antibodies and other cells associated with the immune response.

This will also allow for further repair of the system in general.

When this happens, your body swells around the area.

It will feel warm.

It does not mean that the area is infected yet—it is the area being swollen up to reroute the blood where it belongs.

During all of this, as the immune system is activated and working to function with the body, the cells responsible for the immune system's response will be sending out what are known as cytokines—these allow for communication with the rest of the body.

This is a normal part of the response.

However, cytokines are inflammatory wherever they go.

They can lead to further inflammation of the body if left unchecked.

The vagus nerve, when it detects any levels of cytokines that are abnormal, sends out its own response—it triggers anti-inflammatory neurotransmitters to regulate the immune system's response.

When it does this, it can prevent the body from going overboard—it tells the body to slow down the immune response and stop attacking.

This is done to prevent the body from eventually attacking itself.

Because the vagus nerve plays that role, it is considered very important.

It is responsible for ensuring that the body does not react too strongly to the inflammation that is being built up.

It is encouraging the body to stop being so strong in its assault, either because the response is no longer needed or just to keep the body under control.

Remember, the vagus nerve wants to return the body to homeostasis, which requires the hindrance of the vagus nerve's most common responses, including the response to use this sort of process.

The Vagus Nerve and Healing

The vagus nerve heals more than just the body; however—it can help heal the mind as well.

It is constantly working to ensure that your body is able to heal itself.

It is related to many, many different functions, from the body's sexual response to just being able to breathe.

It is related to inflammation, anxiety, depression, seizures, fainting, and even obesity these days.

Because it is so intricately connected to so much, it becomes incredibly obvious that it is a very powerful nerve.

It is so in tune with everything throughout the body that you must be willing and able to respect the ways in which it will work.

It can even heal the mind, as well.

Not only can you help your body feel better, but you can also change your mindset as well.

You can make yourself feel calmer than ever.

You can help yourself relax when you have been feeling anxious.

It is being used with more frequency in therapies.

People even naturally make use of the sort of vagus nerve stimulation methods that help calm them down.

Just watch someone taking big, deep breaths before they do something that is scaring them—they are triggering the activation of the vagus nerve, which helps them calm down.

The vagus nerve can help with more as well—because it is responsible for that stress response to trauma that either leaves you wanting to fight, wanting to run, or simply freezing up altogether, you are going to have to consider this—what if you are currently suffering from freezing after trauma?

What if you feel so disengaged from the world that you cannot get yourself to do anything at all?

Once again, the vagus nerve can help if you know what you are doing or you have someone guiding you that does.

We will be talking more about the vagus nerve's response to trauma a little bit later in the book, but for now, consider that the body has three responses to trauma—it wants to fight, it wants to run and hide, or it freezes up, and there is nothing that you can do about it.

One of the three will happen in the face of trauma.

Usually, for most people, they are able to regulate out of this.

However, some people never do on their own.

They need to be guided through how they can prevent themselves from panicking, and if you do not guide them through that process yourself, you will find that they are going to struggle further.

They will struggle more than ever trying to better cope with the world around them, or they will simply give up.

However, you can make use of the knowledge that we know about the vagus nerve to help with that as well.

The Vagus Nerve and Treating Epilepsy

Epilepsy is a seizure disorder—it is marked by repeating episodes of the individual's brain activity becoming abnormal.

When a seizure or an episode happens, they are oftentimes found to have sensory disturbances, such as seeing or hearing or smelling something that is not there.

They can lose consciousness sometimes, or at other times, they have seizures or convulsions.

This is all linked to the brain misfiring in some way.

When this happens on the regular, especially with lengthier seizures, it can cause major problems for the person suffering from them.

It can lead to the individual having very real disturbances in their lives.

They can find that they are not able to drive because of the risk of having a seizure behind the wheel.

They may be afraid to go out and about by themselves for fear of having another seizure when they are somewhere unfamiliar.

These very real fears and possibilities can be incredibly disruptive.

Some people can treat their epilepsy with the use of medication.

Some others can use other therapies as well.

However, for some people that have been found to have treatment-resistant epilepsy, it has been found that they can, in some cases, control their epilepsy with the use of a vagal nerve stimulator.

Essentially, these people have a small device that is inserted near their collarbone that is then wired to their vagus nerve.

It is kind of like a pacemaker—it shocks the vagus nerve at certain intervals.

This works by sending an electrical shock to the vagus nerve, which sends impulses to various areas within the brain.

It is not yet known why this is able to treat epilepsy in the first place.

However, people often find that they are able to control the stimulation.

On average, people with a VNS have seen a decrease in seizure activity by 28% in the first three months.
After 6 months, seizures were found to be decreased by 36%.

After 4 years, they were found to have reduced by 58%, and after 10 years, seizures were reduced down by a massive 75%.

While the vagus nerve stimulator is not going to be a perfect cure, it has been found to reduce the frequency of the seizures, with that effect growing stronger the longer the device is installed within someone.

However, the people that have had these devices installed report that they had shorter recovery times in certain situations, and 80% of them reported that they found that their general quality of life had improved.

60% of people reported that they stopped worrying as much about their seizures thanks to the stimulator, and roughly 50% reported that their seizures were not as bad.

This is commonly used when people have found to have drug-resistant epilepsy.

This means that they were not able to get control of seizures after at least two medications.

It is usually used in addition to the medication, rather than alone.

The Vagus Nerve and Treating Depression

Similarly to how the stimulation of the vagus nerve was used with epilepsy, it has also been found to be effective when it comes to treating depression.

It is usually reserved for people that are resistant to other forms of treatment—they must have failed to be able to control their depression with other means, such as with the use of medications or therapies.

When this happens, and the depression is severe, the VNS (vagal nerve stimulator) device is oftentimes installed.

Once again, doctors are not quite sure why this works—they just know that it does.

It seems to relieve the symptoms of depression for those who could not get relief elsewhere, and also allows for people to see an improvement in their life.

Like with epilepsy treatments, it seems to be that the stimulation device requires several months to start working—but it can help you begin to better cope with the depressive symptoms if you have them.

Generally speaking, the doctor will program a dose—the frequency of the jolts of electricity.

Then, you are free to go on your way.

If necessary, there is a special magnet that can be used to temporarily turn off the magnet, and that can then allow for it to be deactivated if there were ever some degree of complication.

Among people that were treated for depression with the use of a VNS, several reported that they felt better.

A study in 2005 followed 329 people that were being treated for depression. 124 got their usual treatment, usually a combination of medication and therapy, and 205 got their usual treatment, along with the use of a VNS device.

They were followed for a year.

After a year, the combination group, the group that received the VNS and their usual treatments, showed more improvement.

27% of patients that did receive VNS showed a significant improvement in their general quality of life and the symptoms that they were suffering form—they reported feeling better than ever.

13% of people that did not get the VNS, on the other hand, reported that they had significant improvement.

This means that between the two, adding the VNS doubled the possibility for significant improvement from depression.

However, as with epilepsy, this is not a rapid treatment.

It takes on average of 9 months to begin to see some sort of response to the VNS actually working, meaning that in some cases, it may simply not be quick enough to properly do what it needs to in order to help other people.

The Vagus Nerve and Treating Rheumatoid Arthritis

Other studies are currently being done on the clinical level that has shown that the vagus nerve, when stimulated, can also aid in the treatment of rheumatoid arthritis, a common autoimmune disorder that people suffer from.

It was found that, in the stimulation of the vagus nerve, either internally or externally, it could help reduce and inhibit the production of the cytokines that the immune system creates to cause inflammation.

This then allows for a reduction in swelling for those suffering from rheumatoid arthritis.

As before with the treatment for depression and epilepsy, this was used to deliver an electrical impulse to the vagus nerve.

In particular, the study being referred to here involved the use of an external device that was held to the neck and then manually activated to deliver the small impulse to the vagus nerve externally, allowing for it to be done without any surgery.

The patients that were enrolled in the study showed significant results that were seen through studies.

They showed a significant decrease in DAS28-CRP—the measurement of disease activity in patients that present with rheumatoid arthritis.

The decrease was rapid—just two days after treatment, they showed reduced levels, and those reduced levels persisted for roughly seven days after treatment.

Pre-treatment, patients presented with an average DAS28-CRP score of 4.19, which showed a moderate level of disease activity.

However, after the treatment with the stimulator, the levels fell to an average of 3.12—enough of a drop to allow the level of activity to be dropped to low.

This is still in the study and trial phase.

However, the results are already looking promising—it is being studied further and developed to allow for it to be honed to a level that can be used on a wider scale to allow for noninvasive treatment of rheumatoid arthritis that will bring a significant decrease in disease activity.

Chapter 4: Vagal Tone and Stimulating the Vagus Nerve

Now that we have established that even doctors and scientists are working hard to make use of the vagus nerve as a method that can treat many different conditions, it is time to begin talking about how this is done.

Generally speaking, the vagus nerve is said to have a vagal tone—the measurement of how well it is working.

This becomes something very important to consider, as we will continue to address within this chapter.

We are going to be looking at vagal tone and how to measure it at first, allowing for an idea of what to expect for the rest of the book.

We will then be spending some time looking at some of the benefits that you can reap when you do stimulate your own vagus nerve.

Finally, we will look at a few of the most common ways that the vagus nerve can be activated to give you an idea of what you will expect for the rest of the book.

Reading this chapter will give you more of the background information that you will need to know in order to understand how the vagus nerve and stimulating it may be right for you.

As you continue through this book, starting on Chapter 7: The Vagus Nerve and the Gut, you will start seeing regular activities and exercises that you can use to help stimulate the vagus nerve to ensure that, at the end of the day, you are able to activate it and reap the benefits that we will see in this chapter.

What is Vagal Tone?

Vagal tone is as simple as the measurement that you will see thrown around for the vagus nerve.

It is essentially the ability that the vagus nerve has to be able to activate and control the body around it.

When you have a higher vagal tone, your vagus nerve is considered to be more efficient, but when it is lower, it is believed to be less efficient.

Considering that your vagus nerve is such an important part of your body and because it does impact so much of how your body is able to regulate, most people want to be able to say that they have a good, toned vagus nerve.

They want to know that their vagus nerve is working efficiently and will allow for the body to regulate better.

After all, if your vagal tone is low, it will not be able to work properly.

Generally, low vagal tone is associated with a myriad of health problems that can plague you.

You can find that your vagal tone, when lower, will lead to many chronic problems that can become very difficult to deal with over longer periods of time.

For example, lower vagal tone is commonly associated with the suffering of chronic inflammation—largely due to the fact that the vagus nerve is the regulator for that sort of inflammatory response in the first place.

It can also cause other problems as well, such as anxiety, depression, and many of the other problems that can be seen throughout the book.
Because vagal tone is so important to develop, you are going to want to practice with it regularly.

In general, if you want to develop that healthy, higher level of vagal tone that you will need to ensure that your body is responding appropriately, as well as to ensure that ultimately, you will be able to heal properly or recover from stress or trauma, you are going to want to be able to work with stimulating your vagus nerve on a regular basis.

If you want to live life with a toned vagus nerve, however, you must make sure that you are engaging with it regularly.

Think of your vagus nerve as a sort of muscle, so to speak—the more you use it, the more toned it becomes, and the more likely you are to be able to cope with the problems that you would otherwise suffer from.

Likewise, when you want your vagus nerve to be toned, you will want to make sure that you are using it regularly to support that healthy development.

Sure, it is used on its own regularly, but some people find that they need a little bit of a boost—they need to regularly stimulate their vagus nerve to keep it up there and working properly.

We will be talking about how to do that regularly in just a moment.

Measuring Vagal Tone

Before you decide whether or not your body is going to have a better or worse vagal tone, however, you are going to need to measure it.

Now, the only way to get a good, accurate measure of this is going to be through the use of invasive procedures that will connect to the nerve to determine how well it works.

Rather than doing that, however, there is a way that you can get a pretty good estimate of your vagus nerve's ability without any sort of invasion.

Many people use what is known as the heart rate variability to determine whether their vagus nerve is toned or not without requiring some sort of invasive procedure that could otherwise lead to future problems.

Rather than doing that, you can instead measure your own heart rate to do so.

All you have to do is track your heart rate while you breathe.

You will want to see what your heart rate is when you breathe in versus what it is when you breathe out.

People with the healthiest of vagus nerves, such as athletes, are going to find that they are able to see a marked decrease in their pulses when they breathe out.

Generally speaking, the larger the difference in your heart rate when you breathe in versus when you breathe out, the better the vagal tone that you have.

This is incredibly easy to do if you have a modern phone—many of them are equipped with a pulse oximeter, which you can use to visually see your pulse in front of you on your phone to allow for a better idea.
However, there is nothing wrong with simply putting your hand up to your neck and measuring that way instead.

Stimulating the Vagus Nerve

If you find that you have a lower vagal tone, you may be wondering how you can possibly treat it—thankfully, there is a very simple answer for you.

All you have to do is make use of vagus nerve stimulation yourself.

You can do this with an electrical device if you could get your hands on one, but you can do it yourself at home as well— without anything at all.

Your entire body is centralized around this nerve, and you are able to interact with it in more ways than you can imagine.

All you have to do is be able to activate it when necessary and then reap the benefits.

The more you do this, the better you will get at it, as well.

When you stimulate your vagus nerve regularly, you will find that, over time, your vagal tone will improve.
This happens naturally—it will slowly but surely allow itself to become better through sheer use.

The more that you use it and the more toned you make your vagus nerve, the more health benefits that you will see over time.

All you have to do is make sure that you use these methods regularly.

Generally speaking, you are going to want to spend time figuring out precisely what it is that you will want to do.

You will need to decide if you want to implement some of the longer activities, such as meditation or other such methods that will better your tone.

However, if you do not want to spend too much time, there are other ways that you can not only support the vagal tone but tone it regularly without much effort.

Even deep breathing exercises while you drive are simple enough to implement without much of a problem and can then allow you to make great use out of your time that you are sitting anyway.

Benefits of Stimulating the Vagus Nerve

When you decide that you want to make use of your vagus nerve, the best way to do so is through learning precisely what you will need to do to better it.

You may find that you are going to find that you benefit in several different ways, depending upon what it is that you are doing.

We are going to go over several of those benefits now, so you will know precisely what you can expect when you begin to stimulate your own vagus nerve at home.

- **You lower inflammation:** One way that you can benefit is from lowering inflammation.

    We have already seen this so far—it was mentioned in the study about treating rheumatoid arthritis.

    When you make use of your vagus nerve to do this, you are ensuring that your body is healthier.

    You can eliminate those cytokines that your body does not need by activating the anti-inflammatory neurotransmitters.

- **You make more memories:** It has been shown in rats that the use of stimulating the vagus nerve can actually strengthen memory.

  In general, it will allow for the release of norepinephrine into the amygdala, aiding in the development of consolidated memories.

  This is also being tested in humans as well as a potential way to treat Alzheimer's disease.

- **You breathe better:** Because you will be activating the release of acetylcholine when you activate your vagus nerve, you will also allow your body to breathe better— the acetylcholine tells your lungs that it is time to take in a big, deep breath.

- **Your body will relax:** As another point to consider when you are using the vagus nerve, you are going to relax yourself.

  Your vagus nerve will trigger acetylcholine, which then tells your body to slow down and rest.

  When you do this as well, many other organs throughout your body release other hormones as well that are related to relaxation and calming down.

- **You recover quickly:** The vagus nerve also works to tell your body to begin to slow down after stress.

  The stronger the response, the more likely that you are to be able to recover quicker.

  You will find that your recovery and return back to a state of homeostasis after a scare or a threat is much higher after the activation of your vagus nerve, especially if you have one that is already toned—this is precisely why people take deep breaths to help themselves regulate their responses.

- **You have better emotional regulation:** Another very common benefit of the vagus nerve being well-toned is emotional regulation.

  When you are able to trigger your vagus nerve during periods of stress, you are able to tell your body to stop when it is stressed out or angry.

  You are able to prevent that stress or that anger response far quicker than other people would use.

  This is precisely why people tend to take in big, deep breaths when they are stressed out—it helps them relax with the use of the vagus nerve.

- **You have better relationships:** As a sort of aside from better emotional regulation, you must also consider the case of being able to better your own relationships as well.

When you are able to regulate how you are feeling at any given point in time, you are able to stop yourself and remind yourself to breathe and relax when you are stressed.

This will then allow you to better make relationships with others.

When you are not blowing up on them left or right in frustration, you will find that you will be a better friend.

However, beyond just that, when your vagus nerve is already naturally toned, you can trust that you will be in that rest and digest a state of calmness much more than you otherwise would be.

Someone who is not chronically anxious, angry, or stressed is going to be able to maintain better relationships in general.

How to Stimulate the Vagus Nerve

Now, if you do have a low vagal tone, it is not the end of the world.

It is strongly recommended that you work on toning it just for your own benefit, but you can do this at home over time with some basic life changes for yourself.

Remember that this is not something that you can just do for a few weeks and then forget about—many of the ways that you can help tone your vagus nerve require long-term life changes.

This means that you will have to allow yourself to better relate to other people.

You will have to spend time working at these regularly.

You will need a schedule that will allow these to be implemented regularly.

If you can do this, you can generally allow yourself to be more prepared and have a vagus nerve that is far more toned than it otherwise would have been.

As you continue to use this on a regular basis, you will find that your vagus nerve will remain strong, much like how you can strengthen and maintain your muscles throughout your body as well to your own benefit.

When you want to stimulate your own vagus nerve, you have a few basic ways that you can do so with relative ease.

For the most part, only the use of electrical stimulation that you will see here will be invasive.

This book will primarily focus on safe, noninvasive methods that you can use to help tone your vagus nerve without causing any sort of side effects or other risks that could be dangerous for you.

If you want to stimulate your own vagus nerve, consider the following methods:

- **Electrical stimulation:** Now, this one will require a doctor, and we will not be discussing how to use electrical stimulation at home.

  If you want to be able to stimulate your own vagus nerve with electricity, you can make the choice to do so, but please consult a doctor first.

While the methods that we will be walking through during this book are generally very low-risk, electrical stimulation can cause side-effects, and it should be discussed with a medical professional before you decide that you are ready to make use of it in your own life.

- **Massage:** Some people like to make use of massage to stimulate their own vagus nerves.

  This is commonly used by doctors, actually—they will massage the neck to trigger a vagal response to allow for the heart rate to regulate itself.

  However, there are other points in the body that you can also use that will trigger a similar response just through this sort of manual stimulation that you can use if you choose to do so.

- **Movement:** Because the vagus nerve runs throughout much of the torso, you can actually begin to stimulate it through your own movements.

  This does not have to be difficult or complex—there are some very simple movements that you will be introduced to later in this book that can aid you through the process of moving just right to pull on the vagus nerve to stimulate it.

  Yoga is the most common way to do this.

- **Sound:** Your vagus nerve travels throughout the neck, and because it is so heavily involved there, you must also consider the ways in which you can stimulate it with the voice.

  Many singing, chanting, and even praying methods can work well to trigger that vagus nerve to get that reaction of calming and relaxation.

  This is precisely why so many people do feel better when they are singing if they happen to get those lower tones that would be needed to activate this sort of stimulation.

  We will be going over several methods to do this as well.

- **Breathing:** The breath is another great way that you can ensure that your vagus nerve remains active and able to continue to become toned.

  There are several different breathing exercises that you can do that will allow you to make use of this.

  You can essentially trigger your vagus nerve to activate if you know what you are doing with your breath.

- **Meditation:** Though surprising to many, meditation actually activates the same pathways in the brain that the vagus nerve does, and you can actually get many of the same benefits.

It is currently believed that the two are more closely related than people thought.

- **Temperature:** The temperature of the air around you, especially with water involved, can also trigger a change in activity for your vagus nerve.

  In particular, oftentimes, people that are exposed to sudden, extreme cold will find that they can activate their vagus nerves.

  They do this often in showers or with a few splashes of cold water to trigger the diving reflex.

Ultimately, there are many, many different methods that you can use to trigger this stimulation of your vagus nerve, and many more exist that have not been mentioned in passing within this chapter.

However, we will see plenty of different options that you will have as we progress through this book.

There are so many options available for you that at least one of them should work well to help you stimulate your own vagus nerve.

Just keep in mind that if you do want to stimulate your own vagus nerve at home, you want to do so while also including the use of a routine.

Try to set up some time each morning, for example, to do one or two of the activities that you will be introduced to throughout the book.

If those work well for you, then decide that it is time to look adding others to your repertoire as well.

You should find that the use of these activities will be well worth the effort as you begin to feel better in mind and body.

Chapter 5: The Anatomy of the Vagus Nerve

Now, before we start getting into how the vagus nerve activates in so many different ways, it becomes important to understand that the vagus nerve exists in two major branches- the dorsal and ventral vagal complexes.

The anatomy of the vagus nerve is very different depending upon which area you are looking at.

As it is so large and travels through most of the body, it has many different features that are worth mentioning and understanding for future reference to ensure that, at the end of the day, you do understand what you are thinking about or talking about at any given point in the system.

We are going to look at some of the major features of the vagus nerve and talk about which kinds of purposes they serve.

This is a nerve that has been developing in life and is found in just about all vertebrates—it is deeply ingrained into our biology and physiology and has evolved over time, expanding upon the more primitive effects that it used to have into the more nuanced, complex response to stress that we have today.

In particular, we will first look at the four nuclei of the vagus nerve—these are major axons that connect to the medulla—the part of the brain stem that the vagus nerve is attached to.

Essentially, there are four strains of the nerve that branch off from the medulla and become what you then know as the vagus nerve.

We will then take a look at both the dorsal and the ventral vagal complexes and the unique features and purposes that each of these areas has on the body.

They serve very different purposes and depending upon which area of which complex is activated, you may find that you have very different feelings and very different tendencies, which is relevant as we move into the next chapter about how the body responds to stress and trauma.

Nuclei of the Vagus Nerve

Before we begin elsewhere, we will first define the nuclei of the vagus nerve.

This is the easiest dividing point of the entire nerve—these are each going to have their own purposes that are all slightly different from the last.

The four nuclei that we will be discussing are the dorsal nucleus of the vagus nerve, the nucleus ambiguous, the solitary nucleus, and the spinal trigeminal nucleus

The dorsal nucleus of the vagus nerve is the part that will be focused on going down toward the organs.

It is directly connected down to allow for the control of the digestive tract and digestive system.

It is a major part of the parasympathetic nervous system in particular.

The nucleus ambiguus is responsible for motor control.

In particular, it allows for control of the pharynx, larynx, and palate.
It also connects to the lungs and heart as well—it allows for the innervation to regulate the parasympathetic system and heart rate.

The solitary nucleus is afferent and connects to the tongue—it allows for taste information to be taken to the brain while also recognizing for sensations within the organs, transmitting it all back to the brain for future monitoring.

The spinal trigeminal nucleus is focused primarily on and around the ear.

This is responsible for the feelings of touch, pain, or temperature with the ear and along with the larynx as well.

However, these are commonly bundled together and thought of instead in terms of being within the dorsal vagal complex and the ventral vagal complex.

To better understand what this means, consider that dorsal means upper or back, while ventral means underneath.

The Dorsal Vagal Complex

The dorsal vagal complex is going to be originated at the dorsal motor nucleus, as the name may have given away.

This is considered the most primitive of the connections that can be made within the vagus nerve.

The dorsal vagal complex has been around throughout time and is unmyelinated.

Myelination is the process by which an axon is surrounded with a myelin sheath—a fatty coating that allows for information to be transmitted far quicker than it normally would without it.

The dorsal vagal complex has precisely one function that it can fall back on.

In times of stress, it freezes—it gains the name vegetative vagus because, when someone goes into this activation, they entirely freeze.

They are overcome with stress and entirely overwhelmed.

They may freeze up and collapse.

They may stop moving.

They may stop thinking altogether.

It is essentially a chance at trying to lose attention from the source that is causing the stress to begin with.

Generally speaking, when you go into a freeze response, it is because the brain does not see any viable option to get out—you cannot fight your way out and you cannot flee safely.

Rather than doing anything and burning through important, valuable energy struggling futilely, this section of the vagus nerve activates and you freeze entirely.

When you freeze up like this, then your body can sort of hold onto all of that valuable energy to use when necessary.

This sort of freeze response will then lift if the threat disappears or if there seems to be a viable escape that you will be able to make.

Beyond just freezing up, this part of the vagus nerve is also responsible for all of the organs beneath the diaphragm—it controls the digestive tract.

This will usually be what causes the digestive tract to slow during any period of stress at all.

This is precisely why people generally do not want to eat when they are stressed—their metabolism has been slowed down to allow for other actions to happen.

The Ventral Vagal Complex

Finally, the ventral vagal complex is the more complicated of the two branches.

This particular branch is a bit more advanced after all of the evolution that has happened since the creation of the vagus nerve.

This is found throughout mammals—it allows for higher levels of cognition and risk versus reward comparisons to figure out how to handle individual stressors rather than simply responding the same no matter the stressor that you are facing.

This activates from the nucleus ambiguus, and will allow you to make a decision when you are confronted with some sort of stress or threat.

Rather than simply freezing up and not moving, your brain gives you two options—you can fight, or you can run away.

No matter which of the two that you choose, however, you are going to have the energy to respond accordingly.

If you want to fight, you are going to feel angry.

You are going to feel that energy that you will need and the adrenaline necessary to help you fight off a threat.

Generally speaking, you will only go into fight mode when you think that you actually have a genuine chance of fighting your way out of the situation that you are currently in.

If you do not have a clear shot at fighting for your freedom, you are going to find that you feel afraid and compelled to run away or hide instead.

You will feel scared and alert, and you will be desperate to find some sort of escape that you can take to avoid any unnecessary attention.

This will be used if you either do not want to fight or you cannot fight back.

It is only if these two possibilities fail, in modern mammals, that they revert back to that freeze response that was discussed in the dorsal vagal nerve.

Within the ventral vagal nerve, you will do anything to up your chances of survival.

The ventral vagus nerve has another major purpose as well; however—it is responsible for any of your social responses.

When you are entirely calm and relaxed, you will find that you go into that proper rest and digest stage.

During this, you feel calm and relaxed, and you are more equipped and able to interact with other people.

It innervates the areas responsible for speech—allowing for communication.

It innervates the ear—allowing for focus on the listening aspect of interactions.

You will also feel more social and inclined to enjoy a social meal or spend time with someone when you are able to use the social activation of your vagus nerve as well.

This is from the uppermost part of the vagus nerve—the part that branches up toward the face.

It is within this area that you are able to activate and control the social engagement system that acts as a sort of honorary third mention within the autonomic nervous system.

We will be discussing these three systems—sympathetic, parasympathetic, and the social engagement system as we go over the response to trauma in the next chapter.

However, for now, be cognizant of the fact that it exists in the first place.

You can make good use of this knowledge, then—and there are many different methods of activating the vagus nerve that will tie into this extra branch that is responsible for socializing.

In particular, smiling is a big one—when you smile and laugh, you can actually begin to activate the vagus nerve to activate those same calming effects, and we will be exploring this as well in the very near future.

Chapter 6: The Vagus Nerve's Role in Trauma

Trauma is an unavoidable part of life. It happens when you least expect it.

It could be in the form of abuse, or in the form of losing someone that you loved unexpectedly.

It could be in being involved in some sort of major accident.

Trauma happens—but the good news is, most people bounce back from it with ease, thanks to the vagus nerve and everything that it does to keep you alive, well, and functioning.

However, sometimes, the vagus nerve does not do a very good job of self-regulating.

Sometimes, the vagus nerve does not activate when it needs to in order to get the mind and body out of the three states of activation during trauma.

Generally speaking, the vagus nerve allows the body to respond one of three ways to trauma when it arises.

It can cause an occurrence of being in fight mode, an occurrence of being in flight mode, or an occurrence of freezing entirely.

You must be able to recognize this in order to understand what happens when things go awry within your own body.

While usually, your body will regulate itself out by activating the vagus nerve and therefore the parasympathetic nervous system to ensure that the body is able to get back to that baseline of normal, it is also possible for the body to never get the hint—it will remain in one of these activations, and that can lead to a whole host of the problems we will be discussing within this book.

What is important to remember, however, is that you can sort of fluidly shift between the mode that your body is currently functioning in, and you can have that shift happen almost instantaneously in some cases.

You are able to see that sometimes, you will go from running to fighting, to freezing, and then back to running.

Think of what happens when you see a mouse being chased by a cat.

The mouse will run as much as possible in hopes of avoiding the cat.

However, if the mouse is not careful, the mouse will be caught.

As soon as the mouse *is* caught, it will freeze—it will stop trying to escape because there is no point in doing so.

If the cat were to let down its guard for just a moment, however, the mouse would take that opportunity and run as quickly as it could to escape.

However, if the cat were to catch the mouse again, it would freeze up once more, locked into that freeze response that we will be talking about shortly.

Your body and mind have to be able to oscillate between the options to stay alive.

Without that oscillation between the ways that it can respond, you get locked into just one default solution at any given point.

However, if everyone simply froze up when someone or something threatened them, it would be much easier to take advantage.

We are going to spend this chapter looking at what it means to say that you are in either fight mode, flight mode, or freeze mode.

Generally speaking, they are all responses to trauma and stress, but they all create very different behaviors and, therefore, must be considered separately from each other.

We will first look at fight or flight mode, and after finishing that, we will take a look at freeze mode to see the difference.

Remember, the default state is the parasympathetic rest and digest mode.

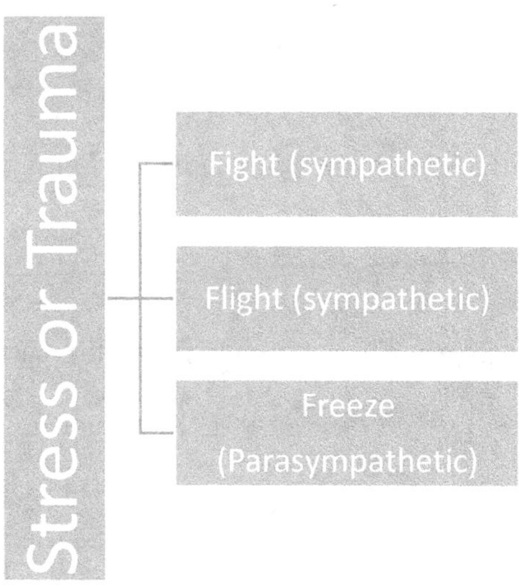

The Sympathetic Response and Fight or Flight

As we have discussed so far, the vagus nerve can lower its activity to lead to allow for the sympathetic nervous system to take control.

With the sympathetic nervous system activated, the body then goes into either fight or flight mode.

These are naturally occurring defense mechanisms that must be considered—when you go into one of these defense mechanism activations, you are going to see that the individual is either going to be ready to fight or ready to run off.

The whole point of this is to keep you alive.

Your body is going to instinctively fight to keep you alive, one way or another.

Without having to think about what it is that you will need to do, your body will snap into action.

You may find that you are pumped to fight—the energy that you will need to help you fend off threats will fill you with that strength that you would need to protect yourself.

Your body will not go into this particular state unless it is confident that it can fight off the threat.

It will do everything in its power to ensure that it can fight off anything that is going to be a real threat if necessary for the benefit of self-preservation.

If you cannot fight off the threat, your body will go into flight mode.

During this state, you feel ready to run.

You want to escape the threats that are in your area so you can survive.

Your mind instinctively decides that running away from the problem is going to be the best possible solution to keep you safe, so it does exactly that—it runs.

Your focus will be on trying to get away from the threat rather than attempting to fight it off.

You may realize that you are not strong enough or well-equipped enough to fight, so you simply do not try to at all.

Typically speaking, as the threat fades away, you will begin to relax.

However, if you do not begin to relax during this stage, you will find that you get caught up in anxiety.

Your body will not naturally unwind, and because of that, you will struggle to see the world without bias.

You will essentially get caught up in that survival mode way of thinking, and because of that, you will not be able to escape the thinking traps that you are otherwise in.

While short-term survival thinking is absolutely essential to life and being able to deal with the challenges that may come your way at some point or another, it is also crucial for you to be able to respond to your surroundings.

Without being able to respond to your threats automatically and systematically without having to think about them, you could run into all sorts of potential problems that could make the situation worse.

You could overthink yourself into inaction, which would ultimately end in not doing anything at all to curtail what needs to be done and in response, you would find that you cannot fend off the threat at all.

When you are feeling the effects of this particular response, your body is in a very stressed stage.

This can leave you feeling exhausted over time, or even like you cannot rest at all.

You will withdraw from socializing and decide that you do not actually want to spend time with others.

This is the activation that was seen in the mouse in the earlier example.

A mouse is not a threat to a cat, so there would be no real way that a mouse could realistically fend off a cat.

Instead of even trying, the mouse focused all of its energy into running away.

By running away, it had the best possible shot at survival just due to the situation in general.

When you are in this sort of sympathetic activation, you normally see or experience the following signs and symptoms:

- Feeling like you are in danger, even if you cannot figure out where that danger is coming from or articulate what the threat really is

- Feeling the effects of stress hormones that will make the body more capable of fighting or fleeing—these are hormones like adrenaline that will allow you to respond quicker and able to move energy and respond quicker.

- Your heart rate will increase, and you feel jittery, restless, or like you need to move around.

  If you are not actively fleeing from someone or something, you may find that you are pacing or fidgeting with something to release that nervous energy.

- You will feel like you are anxious or angry—the anxiety comes from the constant feeling of needing to be alert.

  The anger comes from needing to fight off the response.

  The feelings of fear will come with the desire to run away.

- You will find that your metabolism and digestive system slow down due to the energy being directed elsewhere.

  Your blood and energy are going to be redirected to the muscles to allow for fighting or running—movements that will either help you fend off a threat or run away from it.

- You feel more alert than usual—you feel like you cannot tune out movements, noises, situations, or people because your body is on high alert and focusing entirely on the people around you.

Long-term, this can also lead to feelings of general anxiety.

You are so caught up in the anxiety that you are feeling—that feeling of anticipation that something is about to happen—that you get stuck.

The Parasympathetic Response and Freeze

The parasympathetic freeze response, on the other hand, is associated with hyperactivity of the parasympathetic nervous system.

Remember, the vagus nerve is an inhibitor—it slows down your body when it activates.

When you have an activation of the vagus nerve, you are going to slow down to rest or to relax.

However, when your nerve acts too strongly to inhibit the body and its functions, you can wind up in a freeze response.

Essentially, your mind will dissociate.

You will freeze up and slow down drastically.

This is typically a response that is caused due to the body realizing that it is entirely futile to try to prevent whatever is happening.

Rather than wasting precious resources, you will find that you actually respond by falling into this state in which you do not spend any at all.

If you cannot fight, then the next best thing is to make sure that you shut down entirely.

When you shut down, you are able to conserve that energy that could potentially be used to enable you to escape the threat if the opportunity would arise.

It can also happen, however, when the body is attempting to avoid the trauma.

It is trying to prevent the emotional effects of trauma, so it simply blocks everything out entirely.

This can happen during assaults or during an extreme injury.

The body's responsiveness to the situation diminishes to try to avoid the suffering that would otherwise be endured if nothing were done about it.

People usually describe this as being dissociated.

They say that they are numb—they do not feel as strongly or at all as they normally do.

They may feel like they cannot move or that their bodies are simply limp and do not move.

The body shuts down, so the response will not be as bad.

The body beings to slow—you will usually see a drop in heart rate and a drop in breathing.

At the same time, the digestive system begins to slow, and your cognitive abilities decline.

This is the primitive approach to dealing with threats or traumas—the mind shuts down to try to prevent suffering and pain that would otherwise be endured during a struggle.

If it is truly futile to struggle, this is the best way to avoid it.

The idea is that if you stop moving, you must be dead, and therefore, other attackers may not maintain any sort of interest with you any longer.
If you find that you are suffering from a freeze response, you are likely going to go through the following feelings and experiences:

- You will feel dissociated from your body—you may feel
  dizzy or disconnected from yourself or your body.

  Some people describe it as an out of body experience.

- You may fix your eyes in place somewhere without paying
  any attention to what is there.

  You will not focus on anything.

- Your body begins to slow down—you have a decrease in
  heart rate, blood pressure, and body responses.

  Others will describe you as expressionless.

  It commonly is linked to decreases in sexual and immune
  functions.

- The body's digestive system begins to slow down and
  freeze.

  You may lose control of your bowels, bladder, or vomit in
  response without being able to prevent it.

- Your body will dull its pain response—you will either not
  feel any pain at all, or it will be greatly diminished.

- You will not be able to speak, or you will feel like speaking
  is difficult.

You may feel like you are coking or that you cannot breathe as respiration is slowed down.

- Your brain begins to take in less oxygen as a result of the lowered blood pressure, and this can slow cognition.

  This may be the reason that you see less body awareness or thinking in general.

While some people are able to get out of this relatively unharmed, others can get locked into this sort of shutdown state in which they cannot help how their body is responding.

It may contribute strongly to depression or post-traumatic stress disorder as a result.

Chapter 7: The Vagus Nerve and the Gut

Aside from regulating out the response to trauma, however, the vagus nerve has several other very important functions.

The nerve was, at one point, known as the pneumogastric nerve—pneumo- referring to the lungs, such as when you see the word pneumonia, and gastric referring to the stomach.

This is for very good reason—the reason is that the vagus nerve connects the brain to the lungs and the guts.

Science has shown that your stomach and your mind are intricately related to each other—they are closely related thanks to the vagus nerve.

In fact, due to the high levels of neurons and neurotransmitters that are found within the gut, it is commonly referred to as the second brain—it is the area that you are able to feel things in due to the fact that so many neurons are there.

Of course, there is more to it than just that—the vagus nerve acts as a sort of axis between the two—this axis is referred to as the gut-brain axis and is very important to keep in mind.

When you remember that you have this axis in the body, you begin to see precisely why your gut, the health of your gut, and the presence of certain bacteria within the gut area can actually change the mental state that you are in.

Within this chapter, we are going to discuss the gut-brain axis and why it is so significant.

We will also be taking a look at the vagus nerve and the role that it plays on digestion.

Then, we will take a look at two methods of stimulating and supporting the vagus nerve—with massage and with probiotics that can help ensure that the flora within your gut is healthy and able to support itself.

The Gut-Brain Axis

The gut-brain axis refers to the relationship between the brain and the gut—as the name implies.

This is relevant because your stomach and digestive area are packed with a massive 500 *million* neurons within it.

These neurons are designed to connect to the vagus nerve, where they then act as communication to your brain from your guts.

This is further relevant because of the fact that the bacteria in your guts create neurotransmitters—which your body depends on closely to be able to transmit messages.

They create the impulses that tell your body how to respond.

In particular, serotonin, the neurotransmitter that is commonly implicated in studies on depression and is targeted closely with depression medication, is created not only in the brain but also in the gut.

Within the gut, it directly impacts the act of digestion.

Studies have shown that a disruption of the vagus nerve, whether through stress or otherwise, can lead to stress signals that also impact the guts as well.

In fact, a study done on humans has shown that people with irritable bowel syndrome or Crohn's disease have suffered from reduced vagal tone—it leads to the reduction of function of the nerve, which then impacts the nerve's functionality.

This is a huge problem for people that struggle with their vagal tone—it implies that many of them may actually be at a much higher risk of getting sick than they realized and that can mean that they can very seriously get ill if not treated properly or quickly.

The functionality of the vagus nerve has also been seen further.

A study was done on mice, testing how stress management works.

Certain probiotics, which we will be talking about shortly, are related to the ability to process and cope with stress.

Probiotics are a very important part of keeping the gut balanced and therefore regulating mood, but when you cut the vagus nerve, so there is no ability for the brain to communicate with the gut, and, at least in the studies with the mice, the probiotics for stress management stop working.

This implies the strong effect that the vagus nerve has in mood regulation is related to the gut as well—this means that without a healthy gut biome and without a healthy vagus nerve, mood regulation is going to be all over the place.

The Vagus Nerve and Digestion

The vagus nerve is strongly responsible for the ability to digest your food.

It is directly responsible for all of the movements that will propel your food through your body to manage digestion.

It is also responsible for sending signals from the stomach to the brain that can be used for the regulation of appetite.

When you damage or sever the vagus nerve, depending upon the location, you can wind up with some very serious implications as a direct result.

For example, many people find that they suffer from gastroparesis shortly after the disruption of their vagus nerve.

Gastroparesis is a disorder in which the stomach is paralyzed—they cannot properly push the food from their stomach to the intestines to digest.

This can have very serious repercussions when it does happen—you can wind up with your food, essentially solidifying in your stomach due to this disorder preventing the proper movement.

This can have all sorts of problems—you can wind up with your blood sugar being regulated poorly due to the fact that sometimes, your food will release everything all at once straight into the intestines, causing a sudden spike, while also sometimes creating blood sugar drops even after eating in the first place.

This is a huge problem—when blood sugar is not regulated, there are all sorts of other problems as well.

Some of the most common problems that are associated with gastroparesis include feeling nauseous or vomiting, struggling to eat, feeling full constantly, bloating and pain in the abdominal area, lack of appetite, and weight loss due to malnutrition.

These are huge problems—your body will be unable to feed itself well like this, and because of that, your body will struggle with proper nutrition in general, leading to many other severe problems as well.

Essentially, without a healthy vagus nerve, the digestive tract is going to be crippled as well.

When you cripple the digestive system, however, you cripple the rest of the body as well.

Your digestive system is where your body is able to get all of the nutrition it needs.

Stimulating the Vagus Nerve With Massage

Of course, you can also stimulate the function of your vagus nerve relatively easily—you can do so with the use of an abdominal massage that can be used regularly.

Remember, you can use these methods as often as you would like—however, the more often you do use methods that can stimulate the vagus nerve, the more likely it is that your body will create a toned vagus nerve that you can trust to be effective in ensuring that ultimately, you will be able to support and sustain yourself.

With this massage, you are going to be triggering the vagus nerve through indirect contact—you are going to be pressing on areas that the vagus nerve is present to get the body functioning accordingly.

You can do this relatively easily—all you have to do is ensure that you follow these steps.

1. Begin first thing in the morning—you want to have an
    empty stomach when you use this type of massage to
    ensure that it is as effective as it could possibly be.

    When you make use of this, you are going to want to
    make sure that you lay down flat as well.

    This means that the best time to make use of this
    particular method is going to be first thing in the morning
    before you eat breakfast.

    When you commit to making use of the massage, then
    you will know that your stomach is empty.

2. Slowly, begin massaging and kneading your stomach and
    the abdominal area right underneath the sternum.

    You want to put one hand flat on your stomach and then
    rub downward, straight toward the belly button.

3. Repeat this movement from sternum to belly button with
    both hands in a rhythm, only moving downward as you
    rub.

    As you do this, you are going to want to have some
    pressure, but not enough to be uncomfortable.

4. Then, after a few minutes, you want to change up how
    you massage.

Now, you are going to make use of your fingers to sort of knead at your abdomen.

You are going to want to start at the side near your ribcage.

With circular motions, press gently into your side as you move throughout the body.

Continue to do this as you move down your sides, then up toward the belly button.

Again, this should not be painful—it should feel like pressure without any pain.

5. Lay down and relax after a few minutes.

6. If you so choose, you can move into yoga poses as well that are meant to further encourage the digestive tract, but you can also end it there if that is all you can do.

Stimulating the Vagus Nerve With Probiotics

Because all of the bacteria in your gut directly influence your brain, changing your gut bacteria is believed to be of benefit to people.

Think of it this way—neurotransmitters directly tell nerves to fire.

They tell nerves how to fire to create the right message.

When this happens, they are able to directly alter the way that the vagus nerve and brain function.

With this implication in mind, you do have ways that you can alter the functionality of the vagus nerve, stimulating it to get those same stress-relieving benefits that you would in another way.

The way that you do this is with probiotics.

These are bacteria that will leave you with benefits to your health if you consume and encourage them to grow.

The probiotics that commonly impact the brain are called psychobiotics, and they are strongly effective—they are able to improve stress, anxiety, and depression, all by interacting with the guts.

People who suffer from irritable bowel disorder and anxiety or depression saw an increase in all symptoms when they began to take probiotics.

The catch, however, is that not all probiotics are the same.

In particular, it was Bifidobacterium longum, and it had to be taken for at the very least six weeks before showing improvement.
When you are taking probiotics to help with the brain, however, it is strongly recommended that you also ensure that you are paying close attention to nourishing the bacteria that are thriving within your gut.

You do this primarily with the use of prebiotics.

Prebiotics are the foods that you can eat that will be directly related to nourishing the probiotics that you are trying to foster.

Usually speaking, you will want to dose up on foods high in fiber—the fiber is not something that you, yourself, can digest, but the bacteria that you are trying to foster *is* able to do so.

When the bacteria digests the fiber, it is able to be better supported.

In feeding those good bacteria that need that extra support, you know that you are ensuring that the bacteria has everything that it will need to grow and develop so it can properly support and sustain the health of your vagus nerve.

Essentially, then, you are going to want to be taking a daily prebiotic and a daily probiotic.

Together, you will foster that healthy mix of everything that your body will need to help manage those feelings of anxiety and depression that could otherwise completely debilitate you.

When you can avoid those feelings, and you support your gut health, you know that you are ultimately helping your body to function properly.

You are helping to strengthen your vagus nerve, which you know will help support your body.

There are many foods that can also help you with this sort of support that your body will need in order to develop the healthy gut-brain axis that you need.

In particular, try adding the following to your diet to really help support the body and the brain:

- **Omega-3 fats:** These are commonly found in fatty, oily fish, and they are also highly prevalent in the brain.

  When you regularly consume omega-3s, you are going to increase the good bacteria that exist in your gut while simultaneously ensuring that you are supporting your brain to be strong and healthy.

- **Fermented foods:** Many fermented foods contain the lactic acid bacteria that have also been shown to have great impacts on mood and even tempers.

  In particular, foods such as yogurt, sauerkraut, and kefir can all be found to contain high levels of these healthy bacteria that your body will thrive with.

- **High-fiber food:** The high-fiber foods that you consume, ranging from whole grains to fruits and veggies, will all contain fiber—this is what your probiotics want to consume.

This essentially acts as a prebiotic for those bacteria without taking a special pill, and it has been found that a high-fiber diet actually helps reduce levels of stress.

- **Polyphenol-rich foods:** Foods such as cocoa, olive oil, green tea, and coffee are all full of polyphenols.

  These are chemicals created by plants that your gut bacteria will digest.

  They also typically are found to aid in cognition as well.

- **Tryptophan-rich foods:** Foods that are high in tryptophan support the development of serotonin, that common neurotransmitter that your body needs for mood and digestion regulation.

  Tryptophan is an amino acid that the body uses to create serotonin.

  Foods that are usually higher in tryptophan that you are likely to find include cheese, eggs, and of course, turkey—this is why people usually assume that turkey will make you sleepy on Thanksgiving.

Chapter 8: The Vagus Nerve, Inflammation, and Autoimmunity

Inflammation is another very common problem that people have no choice but to cope with.

When they suffer from inflammation, they oftentimes feel like they have their bodies working against them—and to some degree, they do.

Inflammation is commonly caused by the problems with the reaction that the immune system has.

Usually, the immune system has responded too strongly to something, and as a direct result, you will find that your body is inflamed.

This commonly causes all sorts of issues that can be incredibly painful, incredibly difficult to cope with, but somewhat manageable.

When you recognize that the vagus nerve has been shown to play a role in the removal of the cytokines and other proteins that cause inflammation, you can then see how it is possible to begin mitigating the inflammation altogether if you are able to sort of interrupting it.

You can, essentially, begin to treat the problem, as mentioned earlier in this book.

Within this chapter, we are going to be looking at inflammation and the role that it plays in autoimmune disorders.

They are closely related, and because of that, they are strongly intertwined in terms of how they can directly influence you. When you start to see inflammation on higher scales, you know that ultimately, you are going to see an increase in the potential for the body to begin to attack itself as well.

The body uses inflammation to protect itself, but when there is nothing to protect against, it only does harm to itself rather than ever actually treating it.

Autoimmune and Inflammatory Disorders

It is known that the vagus nerve is related to many of the common autoimmune and inflammatory disorders that people are going to face.

It is commonly recognized that, at the end of the day, people will become inflamed.

However, if the vagus nerve is not able to sort of mitigate that to slow down the inflammation response, it is quite possible that the body will begin to attack itself.

Because the vagus nerve is so strongly involved in releasing those anti-inflammatory neurotransmitters that tell the body to stop, you are going to find that ultimately, the body is not going to be able to function properly without the vagus nerve being strong enough to do so.

The autoimmune disorders that are commonly identified are even broken down into the words auto- meaning "self" and – immune, referring to the immune system.

Essentially, it is an assault on oneself by their immune system.

Evidence has shown that the vagus nerve can treat many inflammatory disorders, such as rheumatoid arthritis.

The people who had their vagus nerve stimulated usually found that they had lower levels of cytokines present as opposed to the people that were not stimulated at all.

This makes sense—the body is going to begin releasing all of those inhibitory effects onto the immune system as well if the vagus nerve is there and active to prevent it from going overboard.

Let's take a brief look at a list of many different inflammation and autoimmune disorders that people are likely to suffer from:

- **Addison's disease:** This disease directly impacts the adrenal glands.

   This is responsible for producing hormones that are used to regulate the body.

   However, when those hormonal balance is thrown out of whack, the body begins to struggle to work effectively.

- **Grave's disease:** This disease is going to attack the adrenal glands.

This leads to hormonal levels being imbalanced, and because of that, you then see problems with the way that the body's metabolism works.

- **Irritable bowel disease:** This happens when your intestines and bowels are inflamed.

  Generally, it is divided into one of two forms—Crohn's disease is defined as anywhere within the digestive tract, while ulcerative colitis is defined specifically within the colon.

- **Multiple sclerosis:** This is caused by the immune system, directly attacking nerves within the body.

  As a direct result, it leads to important nerves being damaged and unable to really be able to manage everything.

- **Psoriasis:** This is caused by the skin cells multiplying too quickly and then creating inflamed skin as the cells multiply too quickly to be kept up with.

- **Rheumatoid arthritis:** This is caused by the immune system directly targeting the joints, then creating warmth, stiffness, redness, soreness, and other discomforts.

  Many people mistake it with normal aging, but it is actually the body destroying the joints.

- **Sjogren's syndrome:** This disorder attacks the body's mucus membranes, leading to problems with the eyes and mouth.

- **Type 1 diabetes:** This is caused by the immune system destroying the cells within the pancreas that are responsible for the production of insulin, which is why there are blood sugar interruptions for these people.

  Without the regulatory insulin in the body, the blood sugar is able to run amok, getting too high and potentially risking damage on the kidneys, heart, and nerves, as well as other areas as well.

Of course, there are many, many more.

Some of these are genetic—they will run in families.

Others are entirely random.

However, no matter why you suffer from it or how your symptoms present, one thing is for sure—you will be uncomfortable, unhappy, and you can usually help mitigate it to some degree.

We are going to take a look at two methods that you can use to treat for these autoimmune disorders that will directly trigger the activation of the vagus nerve and then allow your body to begin to provide that support it needs in mitigating the immune system from overpowering the body.

Stimulating the Vagus Nerve With Cold Therapy

Cold therapy is the use of cold to help activate your vagus nerve.

This oftentimes happens through the use of an ice bath or an icy cold shower, though you could try other methods as well.

No matter what you choose to do, you are going to be stimulating your vagus nerve very easily.

Beyond just that, however, the cold water may actually feel quite good against any inflamed joints that you have, allowing you to then begin to relax and allow yourself to feel better.

When you use this method, you are going to be activating your vagus nerve.

It will then trigger the slowing of your heart rate to conserve energy, and as you do so, your body will begin to slow down as well.

When you do this, you are allowing yourself to also begin producing brown fat, which uses more calories, therefore allowing your body to function better as well.

It will help with the maintaining of a healthy weight that can keep you generally better than ever.

The easiest way you can do this is through the use of a cold shower.
The next time that you are in your shower dedicate the last minute or so to be in the water with it on the coldest setting possible.

It does not take long for you to be able to activate the response with your vagus nerve—even just a few seconds can help.

You will know that you are doing this when you gasp and sort of freeze up for a moment—this means that you are getting the temperature cold enough to have an impact.

When you do this regularly, you will find that you feel like your mind is clearer, that you are more capable of dealing with anything that gets thrown your way, and that your body is able to cope with the inflammation better than ever.

You will want to stay in the water for as long as you can stand, generally speaking, and then allow yourself to get out.

Keep in mind that, while cold therapy can be achieved through just walking in the cold or diving into an icy lake in the middle of winter, this is not exactly recommended.

When you do this, you run the risk of hypothermia—this is dangerous, and many people do actually die when they are not careful in the cold, so you should not expose yourself dangerously or unnecessarily.

Be mindful of keeping safe habits and ensuring that you keep your practices as risk-free as possible.

Cold Therapy

- This involves getting in cold water or a cold situation for a short period of time to trigger an activation of the vagus nerve

Stimulating the Vagus Nerve With Yoga

Another method that you can use to help stimulate the vagus nerve to aid in discomfort and other suffering is the use of yoga.

When you make use of yoga, you are doing so in a way that is going to help influence your body by directly pulling on the vagus nerve.

Remember, it travels throughout most of your body and, as such, will, therefore, be easily influenced by most of your movements.

When you use yoga, you encourage your vagus nerve to be influenced into activating, and in activating your vagus nerve, you start to benefit your body as well.

We are going to take a look at a very common yoga pose that is very, very accessible, no matter your age or flexibility level.

This is a pose of rest—it allows you to mindfully focus on your body and hone your breathing at levels that will aid you in recovering and activating your nerve.

This is known as child's pose—and when you are in this pose, you are going to be on the floor and stretching out your abdomen.

As you stretch out your abdomen, you are going to also be encouraging that nerve to be stretched on as well.

As you do so, it will be stimulated and stimulating; it will then lead to its firing and activating.

This is exactly why those gentle yoga movements are so relaxing and generally uplifting to follow through with—they can really help.

To begin, start on your hands and knees.

You want to keep your back straight while still being relaxed.

As you take in a big, deep breath, you should allow your thinking and breathing to slow.

Feel how the air comes in and out of your abdomen, really focusing on the deep breaths that you are taking.

Then, shift your knees apart.

You will be able to slide down as you do this.

Your toes must be touching here if possible, but if not, allow them to slip apart instead.

Then, lower yourself to the floor.

Now, sit up straight and push up.

You should allow your spine to stretch out. As you do, take in a big, deep breath.

As you do, your chest will expand.

Breathe out and let your body lean forward.

Your hands should stretch out in front of you, much like a cat stretching out, with your bottom and hips raised.

Your palms should rest against the floor, with your knees flat against the floor.

Now, stretch your arms as far as you can and then let them relax for a moment.

Then, pull them back inward so they can rest alongside your torso, pressed against your legs, and allowing the elbows to relax.

As you do so, allow your shoulders to space out, relaxing as they fall and feeling all of the tension fading away.

You will want to remain here for as long as you can or as long as you feel comfortable before you finally begin to end the pose.

Usually, you want to do this for at least one minute before you stop.

When you are ready to leave the pose, you are going to want to slowly and gently walk your hands back to your torso.

Then, you want to slowly position yourself upright and then sit back on your heels.

Yoga

- This involves stretching the body to trigger the vagus nerve thorugh movement

Chapter 9: The Vagus Nerve and Brain Fog

No one enjoys brain fog.

While not a medical condition on its own, it is an experience that many people suffer from and wish that they did not have.

Brain fog can prevent the ability people have to concentrate or to recall memories, and because of that, they oftentimes feel unhappy, unfocused, and generally fatigued.

Generally, people will say that they feel like their thinking is fuzzy—they cannot focus properly, and because of that, they struggle.

Brain fog, like most of the rest of your body, may also be directly related to your vagus nerve.

This means, however, that you are actually able to begin treating it relatively easily if you know what you are doing and how to get through doing so.

All you have to do is ensure that, ultimately, you are taking the time that you will need.

We will be taking a look at everything that you need to know and everything that you can do about suffering from brain fog so you can then begin to better cope with the situation at hand.

Within this chapter, we will first take a look at brain fog itself and then take a look at how it is related to the vagus nerve.

Then, we will look at two more self-stimulation methods that you can use to help yourself hack into your own vagus nerve to help yourself better clear your own thoughts.

What Is Brain Fog

Have you ever been desperate to remember something, only to realize that you cannot figure out what it is or why it was important to you in the first place?

Maybe you felt like, no matter how hard you tried, that though that you wanted to have was entirely out of reach.

You were desperate to remember something, but no matter how hard you tried to figure out what it was, it remained firmly out of reach of yourself.

You could not access the thoughts, and you felt like your brain was slow, foggy, or otherwise difficult to manage.

When this happens, it is usually for a reason.

Though common, it is not normal.

There is some underlying condition that is usually going to result in his sort of discomfort.

The good news, however, is that you do not have to continue to live this way any longer if you do not want to—you can learn to overcome the brain fog so you know that ultimately, you can defeat it entirely.

Brain fog is usually a symptom of another problem rather than the problem itself.

When you are trying to find the source of that disorientation or feeling scatterbrained, you are looking for the source of the problem.

You are looking for the reason that you may be slowing down mentally.

Unfortunately, there are no real easy answers to what causes the brain fog. It could be the early stages of Alzheimer's disease.

It could be from high blood pressure, lupus, or even struggles with sleep hygiene.

However, if you look at several of those causes, ranging from depression, struggles with the thyroid functioning properly, high blood pressure, or other autoimmune disorders that may lead to those symptoms, you realize something—all of those are considered manageable through the use of the vagus nerve.

The Vagus Nerve and Brain Fog

Generally speaking, several of the common causes of brain fog can be related back to the vagus nerve in some way, such as:

- Depression
- Hormonal changes due to thyroid disorders
- Low blood sugar
- Alzheimer's disease
- Multiple sclerosis
- Lupus
- Lack of sleep

Take a look at all of those causes—they can each be related back to the vagus nerve in some way.

As we will be discussing in the chapters to come, depression can potentially be directly related to a parasympathetic shutdown or freeze activation.

We have also seen that the vagus nerve can be used to help manage depression, as we referenced in an earlier study.

Many of the autoimmune disorders we took a look at in the last chapter were also found to attack and target the thyroid, leading to hormonal imbalances that could potentially cause all sorts of other problems that people will have to cope with.

We have also taken a look at the vagus nerve being related to memory and that it is currently being investigated as a potential treatment for people with Alzheimer's disease thanks to the role that it plays in memory management.

Multiple sclerosis is caused due to autoimmune issues as well, leading to an impact on the brain that can be incredibly frustrating to cope with due to it interfering with the way that the nerves are usually able to fire, creating all sorts of further complications for people.

Low blood sugar can be caused due to gastroparesis or other digestive problems, which the vagus nerve malfunctioning can lead to.

Lupus is another autoimmune disorder that wreaks havoc on the entire body, slowly attacking nerves and causing all sorts of problems.

Lacking sleep is a common symptom of the constant sympathetic activation of many people with these problems with their vagus nerve, to begin with.

We have also already looked at how the vagus nerve directly impacts the mind—it is related to the gut bacteria creating the neurotransmitters that are able to activate the vagus nerve.

We saw that in the study, referencing the mouse earlier.

When the mouse took probiotics that are meant to increase mental processing power, you see a lack of benefits when the vagus nerve is weak, damaged, or interrupted.

When you look at high blood pressure as a cause of the brain fog, stimulating the vagus nerve can change that as well.

Remember, the vagus nerve is designed to lower blood pressure when activated, and it does just that by lowering the heart rate thanks to the production of acetylcholine.

With that in mind, it makes perfect sense that the vagus nerve would be implicated in all of it.

This means, then, that the vagus nerve should also be a solution for the problem as well.

If you can activate the vagus nerve, you should then be able to help with clearing the brain in general.

Stimulating the Vagus Nerve With Salivation

One way that you are going to be able to trigger the vagus nerve to activate it is through the use of salivation.

Now, this may sound strange at first—however, making use of salivation is a great way that you can trigger your mind to stop, clear, and begin to focus again through the use of the vagus nerve.

Remember, the vagus nerve is going to activate to lead to all sorts of other effects that will then lead to your mind clearing.

If your problem is that your blood pressure is always too high, this can help you lower it.

If you are anxious or depressed, and that is not helping you either, this can aid in abating those symptoms.

Not only can it help you stop and calm down, but it can also then activate and calm everything else down as well.

The vagus nerve, remember, goes through the face. It innervates the tongue to some degree and also innervates many other areas throughout the body as well.

However, for right now, we are focusing on the fact that it innervates the face.

When you use salivation, you are stimulating the vagus nerve, which is tasked with sending information from the tongue to the brain as a part of its job.

The reason that salivation becomes something important is that it does not happen when you are in any sort of real danger.

Salivation is something that gets inhibited when you are stressed out.

However, when you force yourself to salivate, you will then be able to sort of rewire your brain.

You tell your brain that things must not actually be that bad because you are salivating, and that can only happen when you are not in any danger.

To encourage salivation is actually quite simple.

All you have to do is a simple act of visualization.

When you can visualize what you like to eat, you can then essentially trigger your brain to salivate in anticipation to allow you to then produce that response that you are looking for.

To begin, you are going to take in a big, deep breath and close your eyes.

Think about your favorite food.

Maybe it is a big, shiny, red apple.

Imagine the smell of the apple as you sniff it—that sweetly fragrant scent that smells vaguely tart but sweet at the same time.

Imagine the feel of the apple in your hand as you rub over the smooth, waxy skin.

Imagine the texture of the apple when you bite through the thick, crispy fruit and the juice as it fills your mouth. Imagine the distinct apple taste of the fruit as you do.

You want to visualize it as thoroughly and as realistically as you can to ensure that, at the end of the day, you are able to really imagine what is going on.

When you do this, you essentially encourage your mind to begin to salivate.

You tricked your body into believing that the apple is, in fact, in front of you and that you can, in fact, eat it.

This leads to the salivation effect as you anticipate the fruit in your own mouth.

As this happens, it's important to pool it up in the mouth.

When you allow it to pool up, you will eventually dip your tongue into the saliva and then allow yourself to sort of bathe your tongue in it.

Do this for a minute or two without swallowing- -it is good for you to do this.

Your vagus nerve will then activate.

Repeat this regularly.

This method can actually also be great for you if you are currently having an anxiety or panic attack if you want to make use of it then as well.

- This involves using the body and changing its current state to activate the vagus nerve

Stimulating the Vagus Nerve With Smiles

Another method that works well to trigger the vagus nerve to activate is smiling.

It is theorized that, ultimately, the vagus nerve regulates all social interactions.

When you consider the interactions that the people have with each other are regulated by the vagus nerve, the next step is to consider what it is that makes people interact well with each other in the first place.

Social activity is run by the vagus nerve is nothing new to think about—the vagus nerve, due to the fact that it does regulate the stress responses that people have.

When you consider this, you are going to then think about the fact that activating the social smile is one way that you can then figure out how to begin activating your own vagus nerve.

Not only is the vagus nerve routed through the face, lips, and other general areas of the head, it activates that state of rest and digest, and that is the state in which you are able to socialize with other people.

It is in that state that you know that you are able to really begin relaxing in the ways that you would need to in order to really begin to get that vagal activation.

One major way that you can do this is just with the simple act of smiling—when you smile, you know that you are helping everyone else feel better.

You are ensuring that ultimately, you trigger those good feelings, that vagal activation, and encourage that relationship building a state with everyone else as well.

All you have to do is make sure that you are smiling on a regular basis.

Make sure that you are always smiling at other people.

If you are alone, simply allow yourself to smile on your own, either in a mirror or while sitting by yourself.

You will then be able to really trigger those reactions.

Smiling

• This involves using the body and changing
its current state to activate the vagus nerve

Chapter 10: The Vagus Nerve and Anxiety

Everyone suffers from anxiety at some point or another.

It is an emotion that we all feel to some degree—a simple response to any sort of stress that people are met with.

When you consider this, you are then able to tackle the feelings of anxiety a bit better than before.

However, sometimes, anxiety is more.

Sometimes it goes beyond those feelings of stress or nervousness.

It begins to blend into the territory of becoming disordered instead.

When this happens, it can begin to interfere with your life in many ways that are entirely avoidable, and yet you are entirely enslaved to it without knowing how to stop it.

However, your vagus nerve gives you powerful weapons that you can use against this anxiety.
When you make use of the vagus nerve, you know that you are able to figure out how best to defeat the feelings of anxiety that you have at any point in time.

You are able to learn how to activate your own vagus nerve when necessary so you can then begin to override those feelings of anxiety that would otherwise threaten to rule your life.

Within this chapter, we are going to address the feelings of anxiety and how they are relevant to the vagus nerve.

We are going to go through what is necessary to understand about anxiety itself, taking a look at the common symptoms and then relating it back to the vagus nerve so you can understand the root cause and how they also relate to the parasympathetic nervous system.

Finally, we are going to take a look at two exercises that you can do to sort of eliminate anxiety in its tracks—you are looking at methods that you will know are able to overcome that anxiety and help you defeat it.

What Is Anxiety

Anxiety itself is a feeling—it is the response to stress that drives people to act.

When you are anxious, you feel like you are in danger or that there is some sort of threat.

It could be a threat of physical harm.

It could be a threat of loss.

It could be a threat of just about anything, so long as it is stressful enough to make the individual worry about it.

However, those feelings of stress must also be mitigated somehow to avoid them becoming overwhelming and disruptive.

When you feel the feelings that go along with anxiety, you feel motivated and nervous.

You are going to be antsy and agitated, wanting to figure out how to make that threat or danger go away.

In the short term, that is perfect—it becomes that sort of defense mechanism that you need to keep you alive.

However, in the long term, your anxiety will become your biggest enemy if it goes entirely unmanaged.

Anxiety is going to be a direct result of your feelings—it is going to be coming and going from time to time, but ultimately, it is going to hit you the hardest when you least expect it.

For some people, it is brief.

For others, it becomes a major detriment that needs to be defeated.

Let's go over some of the most common symptoms that you are likely to feel when you are exposed to anxiety.

- **Nervousness:** You are tense or restless, even if you cannot figure out why.

  You feel like there is some sort of danger, or you feel like you are dreading the future.

  You may even have panic attacks directly related to the process that can be debilitating if not regulated properly.

- **High heart rate:** Oftentimes, as the anxiety gets worse, you find that you are suffering from a rapid heart rate.

You are scared and anxious, and this feeling does not help—especially when it is accompanied by rapid breathing and sweating as well.

You may be worried that you are having a heart attack or dying.

- **Twitching:** Some people find that they wind up trembling or twitching in response to their stress or anxiety.

  They are going to be scared of what is happening, and that really exacerbates it.

- **Weakness:** Sometimes, people start to feel like they cannot cope with the situation at hand, and as that happens, they start to feel weaker and lethargic.

  They struggle with their thoughts, and they wind up miserable.

- **Insomnia:** Oftentimes, due to the sympathetic nervous system, insomnia becomes a common symptom.

  Despite the exhaustion felt, they cannot manage their symptoms.

- **Gastrointestinal distress:** It can also commonly lead to problems with your digestive system.

You may find that you have no appetite at all, or you may find that you suffer from vomiting or diarrhea.

Either could happen in response.

- **Avoidant behaviors:** You also commonly may find that you feel a very strong desire to avoid anything that is going to be anxiety-inducing—you will do your best to avoid those problems even if that means that you are going out of your way or disrupting your life to some degree.
- **Feeling out of control:** This is more specific to panic attacks, but oftentimes, people report that they feel entirely out of control.

Despite their best efforts, they feel like they are dying or going crazy at the moment despite trying everything in their power to remain sane, functional, and willing to respond intelligently and rationally.

- **Detaching:** Often, people also feel like they are detaching from themselves and that they are distanced from their bodies.
- **Chest pain and tightness:** Also pretty specific to panic attacks, people report chest pain and tightness as a potential cause.

Anxiety symptoms are oftentimes classified in many different ways.

In fact, anxiety itself is a classification of disorders, not one in particular.

People with anxiety are likely to suffer from:

- **Generalized anxiety disorder:** This is constant or near-constant anxiety about daily activities that are entirely ordinary or mundane.

  Usually, the worry is far more than it should be, and it presents with common physical symptoms such as headaches, nausea, and insomnia.

- **Obsessive-compulsive disorder:** This is commonly known by the constant obsessive thoughts and the rituals performed to try to make them go away.

- **Panic disorder:** This is what people think of when they think of typical anxiety—it is breaking down and panicking in mundane situations.

  It is characterized by repeated bouts of severe anxiety and fear that are unpredictable.

- **Post-traumatic stress disorder:** PTSD is commonly the response to a trauma that is exacerbated.

When someone suffers from this, they do not properly process the fear that they are having, and in response, they may suffer from flashbacks, nightmares, and struggling to relax.

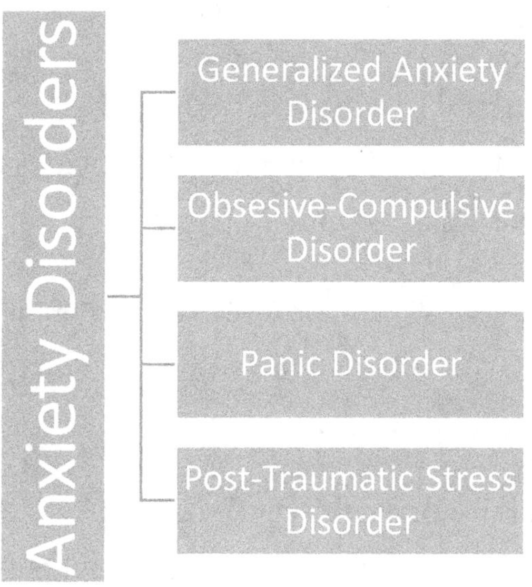

The Vagus Nerve and Anxiety

Remember, the vagus nerve is the sort of ruler and regulator of the autonomic nervous system.

As the autonomic regulator, the vagus nerve has complete control over what you are feeling, why you feel that way, and how you will cope with it.

With that in mind, you must recognize and remember that ultimately, you are going to be bound by your feelings.

They are automatic.

However, just because you are bound by them, and you will feel them automatically does not mean that you must give into them and allow them to rule your life.

Instead, you can spend the time learning to control them—which you can do with the vagus nerve.

When you trigger the vagus nerve, you tell the parasympathetic nervous system to activate.

When this activates, you slow down the focus on the sympathetic nervous system that is going to be weighing down on someone with anxiety.

Instead of then allowing them to suffer, you are able to get ahead of those feelings to overcome them.

You are no longer going to be caught up in the anxiety because you can trigger the body to begin to let go of that particular anxiety instead.

You are able to essentially force yourself to move on past the anxiety so you can begin to act.

When you look at methods that stimulate the vagus nerve, many of them are great for encouraging the body to work the way that it is meant to.

You will see people that are able to do this through breathing, singing, chanting, or anything else that causes that deep, rhythmic breathing.

Think about it—when you were a child, what were you told to do in times of anger or anxiety?

Most people are taught to take a big deep breath because it helps alleviate those symptoms of anxiety or anger, which then allows for the healing of whatever is happening.

You will essentially be able to overcome that anxiety and ensure that instead, you are functioning normally just due to the fact that you will know what you are doing.

You will be able to tap into the body's natural control system to get it to change up how it is responding to the world at large, which will then allow you to better process everything.

Stimulating the Vagus Nerve With Deep Breathing

One way that people commonly defeat their anxiety is through deep, cleansing breaths.

When you breathe deeply, you are able to really begin to clear your mind and your body.

This works precisely like salivating did—you are slowing down the body in order to influence the way that the mind responds.

When the mind sees that your body is beginning to slow down instead of speed up, it realizes that things are not actually that bad—things could not be bad if your heart rate and breathing rate are both dropping so your mind begins to relax as well.

The reason these deep breaths will trigger the vagus nerve is due to the fact that ultimately when you take a big, deep breath, you are altering the pressure within the chest area.

When you breathe in, pressure within the chest cavity drops.

As that pressure drops, the vagus nerve encourages the heartbeat to pick up again to try to offset the drop.

When you breathe out instead, you raise the pressure in the chest to eliminate the air in the lungs.

However, as you do that as well, you are going to see that the vagus nerve again kicks into action.

It is trying to maintain some degree of homeostasis so it activates to drop the heart rate to lower the pressure in the chest by dropping the blood pressure.

It does this because it wants to be able to ensure that your pressures within yourself are staying even and therefore stable.

When you are able to guarantee this, you know that ultimately, you are able to alter your vagus nerve's activity with ease.

All you have to do is know when to breathe and how to breathe.

By far, the most effective simple breathing exercise that you can do is deep breathing.

In particular, it must be diaphragmatic—this means that you are breathing through your diaphragm rather than your chest.

People have a strange habit of sort of suppressing that diaphragmatic breathing rather than utilizing it regularly, and because of that, they then do not breathe in the right way to trigger the vagus nerve in the first place.

To use diaphragmatic breathing, you are going to want to follow these instructions.

Begin by lying flat on your back.

This is more for the first time only just so you can learn what you are doing and how to make it work for you.

You are going to want to ensure that you are lying down so you can pay attention to how you breathe.

Place one hand on your chest and another on your stomach.

As you do this, you will want to pay attention to which hand moves when you do breathe.

If you move your hand on your chest, you know that you are not breathing properly.

If you move the hand on your stomach, on the other hand, you are.

Take in a deep breath with your hand in place.

This will tell you whether or not you are breathing properly in the first place.

After that first breath, and after you confirm that you are, in fact, breathing with your diaphragm, you can then move on to the next half of the exercise.

This can be done in any position that is comfortable for you, and now that you are able to confirm that you are, in fact, breathing that way, you are then able to make use of it.

The breathing exercise that you are going to be looking at is going to require you to do several deep breaths.

Start by breathing through the nose—you are going to need one long, deep inhale through the nose.

It should take you four or five counts as you slowly but deeply breathe in through the nose.

Count the beats as you do.

Then, hold the breath for three seconds.

You want to keep that pressure level in your chest so your vagus nerve will then activate and tell your body to relax to even out the pressure.

Then, breathe out through your mouth.

That breath through your mouth should be nice, slow, and easy.

It should also last for four or five seconds as you let it out, blowing as if you are blowing out a candle.

You will want to repeat this breathing exercise for at least five minutes.

If you can do longer, that is always greatly recommended, but if you do not have five minutes, even just a few quick, deep breaths will make a difference in your general state of mind.

Deep breathing

- This involves using the breath and altering pressure in the chest to activate the vagus nerve

Stimulating the Vagus Nerve With the Valsalva Maneuver

Another common exercise that is done to help with activating the vagus nerve is the Valsalva maneuver.

This is a very particular way of breathing that is going to alter your pressure in your chest.

Just as the deep breathing led to a change in pressure within the chest, you are looking to repeat that here.

You want to ensure that you can raise the pressure in your chest so you can then allow your vagus nerve to trigger and relax the entire body.

This particular exercise was invented in the 1700s by a physician known as Antonio Maria Valsalva, who initially used this as a method of clearing out the ears from pus.

He would use this to change the pressure in the body, therefore allowing for the body to rid itself of the pus.

This method is not very difficult to follow through with.

You simply will want to follow a few quick steps.

Keep mind that if you have problems with your blood pressure, you may not want to make use of this method, but it is generally considered safe for the vast majority of people out there.

You just have to be mindful of how you are going to respond to it if you do make use of it.

To begin, you are going to take a big, deep breath in through your mouth.

Hold it there for a moment.

Then, start to strain your chest and stomach muscles tightly and bear down.

Think of this as if you are straining to have a bowel movement on a toilet—you want that same sort of pressure felt when you use this method.

Then, you are going to want to hold that pressure.

You want to try to hold it for roughly 10 seconds if you can manage to do so.

Then, after the 10 seconds are up, you must force the air out as hard as you can as quickly as you can.

After you do that, you are then going to want to resume breathing as normal.

This will help build up that pressure for yourself to aid in managing your vagus nerve.

If you did it the right way, you will feel the sudden shift in your blood pressure.

Valsalva Maneuver

- This involves using the breath and altering pressure in the chest to activate the vagus nerve

Chapter 11: The Vagus Nerve and Depression

Depression, like anxiety, is an all too common problem that people face.

When you suffer from depression, you are usually quite down about yourself or about life in general—you may feel like you are not worth taking up space in life, or you may feel like other people deserve far better than you.

You may even feel like you would be better off trying to harm yourself because you think that you are little more than a drain on other people.

Depression is one of the most common mental health disorders that people can face.

When you face this disorder, it can lead to you feeling trapped, alone, unable to function, and even wishing that you were dead.

However, there have been great improvements in treatment options for people that do suffer from it.

With that in mind, consider that those treatment options, when nothing else is working, have been the stimulation of the vagus nerve.

Within this chapter, we are going to delve into depression to begin to work out what it is, what it does to the body, and how you can work to defeat it.

When you learn this information, you will better understand what depression is and how it relates to the vagus nerve.

Then, you will be provided with two methods that you can use to figure out how you can activate your vagus nerve to ensure that, at the end of the day, you can actually activate it where it matters the most.

You will be able to do this with ease with the use of these methods.

What Is Depression?

Depression is, at the simplest, a mood disorder.

It leads to feelings of sadness most of the time, while also presenting with a lack of interest in the world.

When you are living life with depression, you will probably have many different disruptions in your own life.

You may find that you struggle with your daily activities or with your emotions at varying points in time.

This is not because you are a problem, but rather because your brain and body are not on the same page.

Depression is not something that you can simply will yourself out of.

You can, however, begin to lessen its effects through many different methods.

You can encourage yourself to defeat it through the use of, for example, changing your diet or exercise routine.

We have already looked at how probiotics have been found to have an effect on mood—one of the ways is in alleviating the symptoms of depression.

When you consider that ultimately, the people that are suffering from depression usually have less serotonin and that is why selective serotonin reuptake inhibitors (SSRIs) are such a common treatment, you are going to recognize that serotonin must play a part somewhere in the feelings of depression—and that is produced commonly within the digestive tract.

When you suffer from depression, you are likely to suffer from many different symptoms, such as:

- **Feeling sad:** You may unexplainably suddenly feel sad, tearful, empty, hopeless, or otherwise despondent
- **Feeling angry:** Sometimes, however, you will feel angry or irritated, even if whatever the problem is, it is not a big deal.
- **Feeling disinterested:** oftentimes, depression comes along with the feelings of disinterest. Even things that once brought you joy are no longer considered exciting or worthwhile.
- **Feeling tired:** Tiredness and sleeplessness are both common symptoms of depression—often at the same time

- **Appetite changes:** Some people report wanting to eat much more, while others do not want to eat as much at all as they used to.

- **Anxiety:** Anxiety and depression are very commonly diagnosed together and are going to make each other worse.

- **Feeling slower:** When you are depressed, you may report that you feel tired, slow, or like you cannot think very clearly

- **Trouble with thoughts:** You may feel like you cannot remember, make decisions, or concentrate very well

- **Thoughts of self-harm or suicide:** Sometimes, depression can make people feel like they would like to harm themselves. This should always be regarded as a medical emergency, and if you ever feel like you want to harm yourself in any way, you must contact emergency services for help to ensure that nothing bad happens to you.

- **Other vague physical problems with no identifiable cause:** People with depression also report that they often feel pain or discomfort for no reason.

The Vagus Nerve and Depression

Go over those symptoms of depression for a moment and think about why they may sound familiar.

If you answered because they are very similar to a parasympathetic shutdown, you are on the right track!

Depression may very well be closely related to the parasympathetic shutdown response that you would see in other people during trauma.

If you think about it, many of them are there.

In depression, people report feeling tired, weak, lethargic, and slow.

All of that happens when the body begins to shut down.

People report struggling to think or make memories.

That also happens commonly during a shutdown when the body is trying to protect itself from harm.

People also commonly report that they do not want to eat at all, which is also in line with the shutdown that people may have with trauma.

While not all depression is going to be caused like this, it may be that treatment-resistant depression is.

We do know that for many types of depression, you can use medication, therapy, or lifestyle changes, but that does not work for everyone.

If you have already tried everything and nothing is working out, this may be the best bet for you—changing to something that you have never tried may be enough to aid in the resolution of your symptoms may help.

While you should never get off of any treatment plant without first discussing with your doctor, you may find that one of these can help you feel better, at least a little bit.

Stimulating the Vagus Nerve With Meditation

Meditation has been found to activate the same parts of the brain and nervous system as the vagus nerve, making it quite effective in managing these symptoms and behaviors.

Meditation is essentially just focusing on clearing one's mind and simply being in the moment.

When you are able to meditate mindfully, you are able to push aside everything else and just focus on what you are feeling at the moment so you can live by that moment at the moment.

It does not have to be difficult. You can meditate very easily if you can follow these steps.

First, begin by finding yourself somewhere comfortable.
It should be somewhere that you know that you are not going to be distracted for a few minutes.

At first, try to set aside at least 5 or 10 minutes, but if you can get your time up to at least 15 minutes in a session, you will see the best benefits from this.

When you are comfortable, sit back and take in a deep breath.

Clear your mind.

Allow yourself to focus entirely on your breath as it comes in.

Remember your deep breathing exercise and use it here.

Then, breathe out.

You want to set up your breathing to be in 5 second intervals—5 in, 5 out.

This will give you the best possible impact of this particular exercise.

You must also ensure that you are focusing entirely on your breathing.

Do not pay attention to anything else around you, and any time your mind wanders, correct it gently back to the task.

You will return it back to yourself so you can continue to meditate effectively.

Do this for at least 5 minutes, but for as long as you have available.

Try to make this a daily exercise for yourself if you can make it work for you.

- This involves calming the mind to activate the vagus nerve

Stimulating the Vagus Nerve With Bee Breathing

Another common exercise that people will use to stimulate their vagus nerve is known as bee breathing.

When you use bee breathing, you are going to be focusing on how you breathe to trigger your vagus nerve to activate for you.

You will essentially be building up pressure within your body and breathing loudly to sort of stimulate your vagus nerve.

In particular, this will involve stimulating the vagus nerve in the throat—particularly in the vocal cords.

When you activate your vocal cords, you vibrate the area, which turns on the vagus nerve.

To begin, sit down and get comfortable.

When you are there, you can then begin to interact with your vagus nerve effectively.

You are going to want to straighten your spine and then take in a big, deep breath.
Then, close your eyes for a moment.

Seal your lips as tightly together as you can so no air can escape, then take in a deep breath through your nose.

As you do this, you are going to want to hum the sound of the letter M.

You want to make a long, loud, "Mmmm" sound to really get this particular exercise down.

As you do this, you are going to want to cover up your ears with the palms of your hand.

You will do this for as long as you can muster before being done.

Keep in mind that you are not trying to push yourself here—you should simply do it for however long you enjoy before moving on.

Bee breathing

- This involves using the breath and vibrations in the neck and in the chest to activate the vagus nerve

Chapter 12: The Vagus Nerve and Other Common Conditions

At this point, we are going to look at a few more exercises that are commonly related to the vagus nerve and then two more methods that you can use to help activate your vagus nerve.

In particular, we are going to address gastroparesis in a bit more depth here, and we are going to talk about syncope and what it is.

Finally, we will touch upon the link between the vagus nerve and obesity.

And then, we will look at how both singing and laughter can be used to activate the vagus nerve and really help with the stimulation.

Other Common Conditions

Gastroparesis

Gastroparesis, as we have looked at already, is the paralysis of the stomach due to a problem with the vagus nerve.

It commonly happens in response to some sort of damage to the nerve—it could have been severed in surgery, for example, or it could have happened some other way.

When it happens, however, the vagus nerve is no longer able to communicate with the stomach to tell it to get moving when it is lagging.

This is a problem; however—it can lead to further problems when no food is being transferred through the digestive system.

Syncope

Syncope is the diagnostic name for fainting.

If you faint, you have had a syncope.

These are not generally dangerous, but they are usually considered related to the vagus nerve's response to stress or something else that has caused anxiety or trauma.

When you have a syncope, you are going to find that your blood pressure suddenly plummets.

This happens to try to protect the individual but oftentimes ends instead of causing other problems.

Rather than activating properly, the vagus nerve goes overboard and causes your blood pressure to drop, and without adequate blood flow to the brain, you will naturally lose consciousness.

Obesity

Current research is linking obesity with the vagus nerve as well.

Researchers are connecting the way that the vagus nerve regulates itself out to provide feedback to the brain as a potential reason for obesity.

If the vagus nerve does not communicate properly, there are going to be other problems that arise, and because of that, it may be related to far more than just paralyzing the stomach.

Since the vagus nerve is supposed to tell the brain when the stomach is full, it failing to do so could be linked here.

Currently, experimentation is being done to see if the vagus nerve has any potential as a key to treating obesity in people.

Singing to Activate the Vagus Nerve

One way that the vagus nerve can be activated is through song.

Generally speaking, if you are going to sing to activate the vagus nerve, you must do so with a deep, throaty voice as you do so.

You are going to want to trigger those big vibrations throughout the throat to trigger the stimulation of the vagus nerve.

Like the use of the bee breathing exercise, this will make use of the fact that your vagus nerve is intertwined with the vocal cords, and therefore, you can activate them within each other.

If you want to sing, you can pick out just about anything—really, what matters here is that you have to like it.

It can help as well that when you sing, especially if you get really into it, you are going to find that your breathing is deeper.

This makes sense—you have to pull in a lot of air to sing, especially if doing so loudly or passionately.

With that in mind, consider the fact that sing becomes a great way to help.

While you may not be able to sing freely everywhere and anywhere you go, you do have many areas where you can do so.

You can sing, for example, in the car on the way to work when you know that you have a very stressful meeting coming up.

Instead of stressing, you have some fun, and you activate your vagus nerve while you do it.

Singing it out, then, becomes a great, enjoyable, and versatile way to make use of your vagus nerve and your biology.

> **Singing**
>
> • This involves using the breath and vibrations in the nect to activate the vagus nerve

Laughter to Activate the Vagus Nerve

Finally, laughter is another fantastic method that is enjoyable and can also activate the vagus nerve.

Remember, the vagus nerve is intertwined with the areas of your body and mind that are responsible for socialization, and because it does relate to that social aspect, which can only happen under a parasympathetic state of being at rest, laughter becomes a great method that you can use to stimulate your vagus nerve and help yourself and others begin to feel better.

All you have to do is ensure that you are spending the time that you otherwise would laughing.

You can start by laughing in private—even fake laughing is good enough here.

The idea is to get your body moving in this manner, much like how you fake smiled to trigger a real smile or how you thought about an apple to make yourself salivate for one.

When you are able to laugh at yourself and laugh with yourself, you are then able to ensure that you activate your vagus nerve with ease.

All that matters here is that you spend the time to laugh.

This is why you always feel so good after a good laugh session.

If you have not laughed in a while, you are now challenged to go out, find a funny movie, and spend the evening watching it.

You may find that you love and enjoy doing so, and you will activate your vagus nerve at the same time. That is a win-win situation!

- This involves breathing, vibrations in the neck, and social engagement to activate the vagus nerve.

Conclusion

Thank you for making it through to the end of *Healing Power of the Vagus Nerve.*

Hopefully, it was informative and able to provide you with all of the tools you need to achieve your goals.

Within this book, you were guided through everything that you would need to be able to activate your own vagus nerve and how to make better use of it.

You learned all about how your vagus nerve works, looking at it within the nervous system itself and then exploring how it benefits the body.

You have gained the knowledge to check if your own vegas nerve is toned and able to regulate your body or if it is likely causing issues for you.

You now even have the knowledge on how to work to stimulate and tone your vagus nerve.

You spent time learning about the autonomic nervous system—
the part of your nervous system that controls everything out of
your own conscious access.

You learned about how the vagus nerve is able to heal and exactly
how you can use the vagus nerve to heal yourself as well.

From here, all that is left for you to do is begin making use of this
newfound information.

If you believe that your vagus nerve may be weak or strained,
there is no time like the present to begin understanding why that
is the case.
You can learn everything that you need to know about yourself
and how your vagus nerve activates your body with ease, so long
as you are willing to spend the time doing so.

Thank you so much for taking this book with you on your journey
into discovering your vagus nerve and how it works for you.

In reading through this book, you were introduced to a very
magical, underappreciated part of your body that actually
regulates out most of what you do—it is incredibly valuable to
recognize what the vagus nerve can do for you, and you now can
do that.

You can now begin to tap into the healing power of the vagus nerve to activate your own vagus nerve to overcome so much of the struggles that you may face on a regular basis.

Whether you are chronically ill, overstimulated, stressed out, depressed, anxious, or otherwise struggling, these techniques will hopefully help you find peace and comfort, no matter what the reason is for your struggling.

Finally, if you found this book useful in any way, a review on Amazon is always appreciated!

List of Books written by Dr. Louise Lily Wain

Chakra Healing For Beginners: A Complete Guide to Awakening, Clearing, Unblocking and Balancing your Chakras and Your Life Through Guided meditations, Crystals, the Power of Affirmations and Yoga

Reiki Healing for Beginners: A step-by-step guide to Heal your Life, Improve your Health, and increase your Energy. Reiki

Guided Meditations, Distance Healing, Working with Crystals and on Pets

Empath Healing : A survival guide to Stop Absorbing Negative Energies and Healing from Emotional Manipulation and Narcissistic abuse. Become an empowered empath by strengthening your own empathy

Master Your Emotions: Rewire Your Mind, Manage Your Feelings, Overcome Negativity, Reduce Anxiety, Stress, Anger, Worry, Develop Self-Control, and Live a Happier Life

Emotional Intelligence for Leadership: Improve Your Skills to Succeed in Business, Manage People, and Become a Great Leader — Boost Your EQ and Improve Social Skills, Self-Awareness and Charisma.

How to Analyze People: The art of reading people, discover various personality types and patterns, understand human behavior, learn types of body language and how to refrain from manipulating people.

Influence Human Behavior: Mind Control Techniques and Principles of Persuasion to be more likable, more persuasive, more confident, win friends, influence people and avoid manipulation

www.ingramcontent.com/pod-product-compliance
Lightning Source LLC
Chambersburg PA
CBHW070657250726
48662CB00001B/173